# JENNIFER MAY

# Pure Health and Happiness

*8 Weeks To Change Your Life*

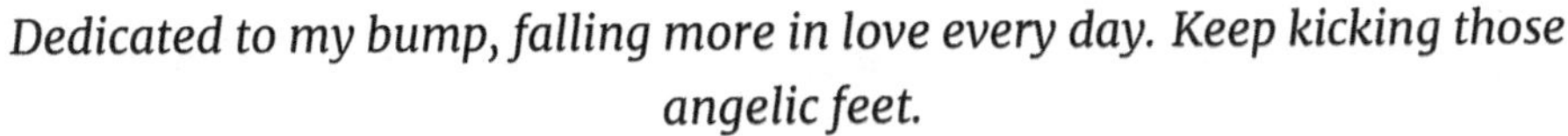

*Dedicated to my bump, falling more in love every day. Keep kicking those angelic feet.*

*To Paige, Lexi and Damon, for teaching me what unconditional love means.*

*To my Mother, Brother, Grandmother and Katy for your endless love & support.*

*To Riaz, for loving me when I didn't love myself*

*Thank you*

# Contents

## VII   Week 5: Reducing anxiety & stress



## VIII   Week 6: Building better energy



## IX   Week 7: Your guide to exercise



## X   Week 8: A low-tox life

XI    Post-program health, happiness & achievement assessment



XII    Recipes

# I

My story & how we're going to change your life

# Introduction

I knew I had hit rock bottom when I lay in my hospital bed praying for a diagnosis that meant I would have to be admitted. I'd visited this particular hospital three times in the last two weeks, only to be sent home again shortly after. This time I could barely breathe, barely stand, I felt as if a large blade was tearing open my lungs with each laboured breath.

After being told to leave once more, I lay in my hospital bed sobbing silently. Desperate, pathetic whimpers - all I was capable of.

Moments later the doctor returned and found that I (luckily) had not yet left, I was told that my blood tests had proven that I had pneumonia and septicaemia. I would need to stay in the hospital for another week or so at least. If my lift home had arrived sooner, I may not have made it through the night. I didn't know it yet, but the incompetence of the medical staff at this hospital would fuel a drive and dedication to helping others for years to come. Ultimately this would change my life forever.

For now, however, all I could think is that I had never felt more relieved. Relieved that there was actually something medically wrong with me - a justification for why I felt so awful. Relieved that my emotional overwhelm and physical exhaustion had a cause... it wasn't all in my head after all. Most of all I was grateful that I had medical approval to lie in bed and convalesce and, importantly, I would not go home to that house... at least for a couple of weeks.

The year was 2003. I was 21 years old and sicker than I'd ever been, yet I'd felt unwell for as long as I could remember. Back then I had no idea what it felt like to be happy, healthy, to have energy, real energy, not the type that came out of a can of energy drink. I would discover years later how easily I could have turned my life around right then. How much healthier and happier I could have been, just by changing my diet.

I had abused my body, my mind and my privilege to a peaceful adult life. I kept bad company, ate bad food (think instant noodles, cans of macaroni and cheese, on a good day though I'd head to KFC and have a Zinger Wrap, yes that believe it or not was a healthy day).

I drank too much, I stayed up all night and stayed in bed all day whenever possible. I was an unhappy, unhealthy young woman and my body was beginning to shut down.

I had been fatigued and depressed for so long that I genuinely did not think it was possible to feel any other way. I did not enjoy being alive, rarely got out of bed before 2 pm and never, ever, woke to feel rested. I had no idea how to help myself, and neither did my doctors – and yet it was all so simple.

Nine years later, in 2010 and in the final year of my studies of Nutritional Medicine, was where I learned what had been missing all along. I'd been pushing myself too hard once again, working 2 jobs and staying up all night finishing assignments, relaxing with a bottle of gin or wine, comforting myself with junk food and telling myself I could get away with it.

Here's where the final push came. After temporarily losing my vision to a tumour on my retina and being treated with a chemotherapy drug injected into my eyeball (while conscious I must add), I would experience first hand the incredible power of food. I put in to practice everything that I'd learned throughout my 3 years of study and knuckled down and set myself a strict regime that turned out to have seriously powerful effects. I turned my whole life around in just 8 weeks. I got my vision back, and along the way gained better health, happiness and vitality than I'd ever thought possible.

Fast forward to 2018. I am a Nutritionist with two successful businesses and a healthy, happy life. My friends now appreciate my values and encourage me to be the best version of myself. My family is proud of me and, for once in my life, I agree that they should be. And most importantly of all, my once diagnosed "possibly infertile" self is currently growing my first beautiful baby and though I'm supposed to be tired (apparently), I've honestly never felt better.

I'm excited to share with you the tools I used to turn my life around and gain the health and happiness we all deserve. The changes I made to my diet and lifestyle gave me the strength, confidence and energy to push forward and turn my whole life around. If only I had known the power was right there, at the end of my fork.

I will summarise what I learned from my personal journey, my studies, my clinical and personal experience, and my patients' success stories to give you a step-by-step formula for achieving your highest level of health and happiness. I am going to work with you to get you on your way to changing your life for the better, for good.

Give just eight weeks of your life to this program and commit to it wholeheartedly and you too can change your life. I promise you are capable of more than you know and will be surprised at how much healthier, happier and more energised you can be when we introduce some simple diet and lifestyle changes.

This book is for anyone who wants to improve their health and well-being, their sense of purpose, their energy levels and their zest for life.  If you would like to be the best possible version of yourself; to enjoy fitness, to look forward to playtime with the kids, to become something greater than your life seems to have destined you to be. Break free from the trappings of your fate, and push forward with a fierce and unwavering determination for unfiltered undiluted happiness and health.

Moreover, if you are currently overworked, overweight, over-whelmed and ready to pack it all in, I am here for you. If you view healthy, happy people as some out of reach, elite, secret society to which you are excluded, I get it. I was on the outside too. Now my life is dedicated to the health transformation of others. Over my years of practice I've developed and perfected a transformational health assessment called the Comprehensive Health Screening. This addresses all of those areas we often let slip during busy, stressful times. I assess a person's current and future well-being based on their diet and lifestyle practices, along with their hormones, toxicity exposure, stress levels, and energy. From here I map out an 8 week plan for them to transform their life step by step to achieve Pure Health & Happiness.

I could not have conceived this method without recognising my weakness and my failings to take care of myself. This has now allowed me to help countless patients. I've poured as much info and support as I can into this book to help you turn your life around. For those of you who'd like more guidance, or if you'd prefer an individually tailored version of this program, head to www.sydneycitynutrition-ist.com/shop and book your Comprehensive Health Screening.

# Where It All Began

In my early 20s, I was unhealthy in every possible way. My relationship was physically and mentally abusive, I had no purpose, I was exhausted and unhappy counting down the days to the weekends where I could drink my troubles away. Week after week I became more depressed, more emotionally and physically exhausted. My current lifestyle was swallowing me whole, and I needed to get out.

Then came my trip to Ibiza. Like many 20 somethings, I partied all night, and by day I went to boat parties, bar crawls, booze cruises and occasionally slept (usually on the beach in the sun). I pushed my body to the limit. This life was coming to an end, though I did not know it yet. My body had decided it had had enough; it was ready to shut me down, force me out, change or die - the latter was closer than I realised.

On the plane journey home I would stop breathing, delaying the whole flight for all the other irritated passengers who gossiped and rolled their eyes as I felt equal parts shame and panic. "Please don't let me die here." I thought, "That would be so... embarrassing".

How did I end up here? Well, life up until this point had not been great. My youth was not privileged or peaceful. I stopped being able to show any real emotion at age 11 after seeing my mum devastated when my father, the love of her life, had just decided to leave us again

3 days before Christmas (he'd been absent since I was 3 months old). This was particularly devastating as this time spent with my father was the first time I'd seen mum truly happy and at peace.

Even at that young age, I had never blamed my father for his absence, despite the fact that this had led to a ripple of events and interactions that had left lasting lifelong scars.

However I'd come to feel more stable and secure with him around. He was a positive role model and I felt safe with him. Now that he was leaving (again) my trust in people was completely shattered.

When my mum announced her cancer when I was 13, my world imploded. The one constant in my life was now threatened. I spent my 14th birthday alone contemplating the worst in my new stepfathers home, while my mum had surgery. She recovered thankfully but her health struggled for many years to come and we had many major scares.

My mums experience while in the hospital was terrible. You could say that the experiences she had were the primary fuel for my resolve to change the health, (and health-care support options) of the world.

However what I didn't understand at that time was that through all my stress there was an underlying drain on my nutrient reserves that was further driving my depression, fatigue and exhaustion. This led me to accept a life far less than I deserved for far too long during my young adult life.

The physical consequences of stress are incredible. In traditional medicine, we call stress "The Great Undoer". In prolonged, severe stress and trauma, particularly during childhood and developmental years, these consequences are more extreme, more threatening and, unfortunately, take a lot more time and effort to counterbalance. Not that I tried until many years later.

Like most people, I had no idea at all how much a healthy diet and lifestyle could change my life. I would never have believed if you'd told me that I could wake up with energy, could exercise regularly without always injuring myself or that I could feel happy and confident in my skin and have the drive, determination (and energy) to help thousands of people live healthier, happier lives.

It took me years to finally step up. Years of hard work, a few lucky turns, some beautiful supportive and positively influencing people and finally, fearing the loss of my eyesight before I was ready to make the change. Through all of this, my thirst for knowledge drank up every last drop of learning and experience which would further my ability to heal myself and others. I have discovered what is necessary, what is helpful and what is just a plain useless waste of time.

I have developed a step by step process, which I have put into practice in my life and my work with my patients. My work with my patients is now to support a whole health overview, working towards a better life, rather than simply changing how we eat. Most of all I have developed a compassion that can only be gained by someone who has walked in the shoes of an exhausted, unhappy and unwell human being for many years.

In this book, I will take the eight key elements which turned my life around and which continue to enrich and empower my patients and my own health to this day. I will lay out a success formula for healthy, empowered living that you can easily achieve, easily maintain and which, if followed correctly, will offer you quick and long lasting results.

If you are serious about changing your life, then you and I will work together through the pages of this book to fill you to the brim with the knowledge and experience that took me a lifetime of learning, dedicated study and years of professional practice to discover. Together we will form the fabric of your new life and work towards that younger, stronger, happier you. Are you ready?...

# Where We Are Heading

So now you know the beginning of my story, the jagged pieces of me that once had me feeling broken but now make up my determination, my resolve and daily drive to help others live a happier, healthier life.

If you have picked up this book you're likely looking to turn your life around. I'm here to take away the overwhelm and help you focus on what really matters, step-by-step.

No matter where you are right now, no matter how broken, jaded, exhausted or overwhelmed you are, I promise you there are some simple diet and lifestyle changes which can help you feel like that younger, stronger, happier you.

Don't worry if you're currently feeling too exhausted to make any change.  If this is how you feel then for now just feel good about committing to reading. Feel free to read through chapter by chapter in your own time. When you feel ready, take on any task from the weekly to-do lists that excite or interests you. With your new found knowledge you'll no doubt be making healthy changes habitually, with very little effort and sometimes without even realising it. As your energy improves you'll feel ready for more change.

Each week I'll be adding new steps and focus points. You'll learn why each step is important and how to implement each step into your daily life. Then I'll provide a to-do list. Each week you'll also find that there are tips and tricks for those who don't have the energy or time to commit to all steps.

This book is a whole health overhaul built on a foundation of my studies in natural medicine and health science, my personal real-life experience and thousands of clinical case studies from those I've worked with over the years. I am pouring my blood, sweat and actual tears into these pages to give you real and practical to-do-lists that will affect real change.

I've travelled my journey, I took many wrong turns and was distracted and derailed more often than someone losing badly at a game of snakes and ladders.  In the end, though, I arrived where I am today. I'm now happy, I'm healthy and I'm working hard every day to positively affect the lives of others. You are no exception, you are my mission, your health, happiness and vitality are my goals. Thank you for this opportunity!

# Who Needs This Book

I'm going to ask you a question. Do you consider yourself healthy? Do you feel happy? Do you find yourself in control of your energy levels, mood, weight, hormones, cravings? Are you achieving all that you set out to achieve? Or are you finding yourself feeling overwhelmed and out of control?

Also, what does healthy look like for you? Are you in perfect health right now? Is there more you could be doing? Are you experiencing the full fruits of your labour?

Maybe your life, your health and your happiness are all at their peak right now, if so then I hope to offer some new insight into how to keep it there. Health is too precious to take for granted.

For those reading this however who are battling fatigue, stubborn weight gain, chronic anxiety, depression, insomnia, chronic sickness, unbalanced hormones, PCOS or other lifestyle-related illnesses, this book is for you. For those who are just ready to feel entirely utterly awesome, this book is, of course, for you.

I want to be here for you, I want to journey with you, I want to take your hand and tell you YOU CAN DO THIS. I want you to say to yourself that you deserve more. I want to hug out your insecurity, beat out your stubborn resistance, fill you up with knowledge, health and happiness until you can no longer contain yourself, you'll need to tell everyone you meet.

In week one we are laying the foundations for all that we are about to do. I am a firm believer that we cannot begin our journey towards reaching our goals until we truly understand our starting point. From here we will plot the beginning, sketch out the destination and map out the route which we will travel for the next eight weeks together.

Now no more dilly-dallying. I am dancing around here on my tippy toes like a kid at Christmas. Overflowing with urgency to get stuck into the meaty bit of this book - the Pure Health & Happiness method.

Are you with me?... Let's change your life...

# II

# Getting to know you

# Getting to Know Your Preferences

In an age where media airbrushing and social media highlighting has blurred the lines of individuality, we often forget to get in touch with who we really are. What stimulates you? Uplifts you? Motivates you? What makes you feel happy? What makes you feel calm? Equally important is knowing what makes you feel angry? Passionate? Anxious?

By understanding these things, we can begin to change our environment, our comfort spots, our retreats and our daily habits to form a more centred, calmer, happier and healthier version of ourselves. We can also be sure to set achievable goals that are true to our core needs.

Let me give you an example:

I am very stimulated by colours, light and sound By understanding this I can make the most important decisions based on what will preserve my health and happiness.

When choosing where to live, I will select a sun-filled home, with a great view, filled with sounds which calm me and which has the sunrise filling my home with light each morning, helping to balance my sleep-wake cycles.

I will choose these factors over the location, the size or even the price of my home as this means it is my sanctuary. I can go there to recharge, can wake feeling energised by the light of each day and can gaze out at my beautiful view filled with all of the beautiful colours that I find so spiritually and emotionally uplifting.

The prestige of a location would not provide me with equal benefit unless it also offered the light, colour and sounds I crave. If I was to live in a home which was dark, crowded and filled with the wrong kind of sounds then I could easily and quickly become fatigued, unmotivated and depressed. I made this mistake a few times before I made the effort to get to know myself.

When choosing a clinic location, the colours and natural light are again highly significant. Being a Natural Medicine Practitioner is not all smiles and gratitude. It can be tough to wholeheartedly give your inspiration, knowledge and passion to uplift and revive person after person whom themselves are feeling fatigued, depressed, overwhelmed or even empty. I need to be filled to the brim each day, with energy and inspiration to spare, allowing me to "give from the overflow" as Alexis, one of my lovely interns puts it.

I'm also a textural eater meaning that the texture of my food is as important (sometimes even more important) than the flavour of my diet. I don't like foods which are rubbery or those which expand in your mouth as you eat them. Foods such as calamari or octopus, for example, are very much out for me. Understanding this, I place equal importance on the balance of textures in my meals as the flavour which means my healthy meals are enjoyable. My salads can be as satisfying as tucking into a slice of cake (sometimes even more so) because I've taken care to balance textures and flavours.

Understanding yourself in this way allows you to use this information in your favour. Let's get these preferences working for you not against you.

# What Stimulates You?

W hat gets you going even when you've had little sleep or are feeling flat (coffee does not apply here)? What lifts you up? Makes you feel excited or passionate? What gets you moving? This can be an idea, a workspace, a type of lighting or particular sounds. It may be music, your favourite cafe, a kind of interaction or even a specific movie.

Over this next week, we are going to be taking stock of the nitty gritty parts of you - the individual pieces that make up this beautiful puzzle that is your unique being. I would like you to carry a notebook and start writing down any glimmers of happiness, motivation, excitement or energy. Take note of from where this inspiration came, if you are not sure, just note the feeling and the location and events that led to this feeling. Over time patterns will emerge, and you will begin to understand yourself a little better. This is just the beginning of the journey to the stronger, happier, healthier version of yourself that you may currently feel is out of reach.

For example: knowing that bright light stimulates me, I know to work in bright spaces when I need to be uplifted and energised. However, it also means I know that I need softer lighting to be calmed or go to sleep. Before understanding these things, I would often find myself overstimulated and overwhelmed - buzzing with energy and ideas at midnight and wanting to rest when it was time to rise, and usually, I'd see myself struggling with motivation to get essential tasks done.

As a result, I was always under-rested and over-stimulated. I relied on caffeine through the day and regularly needed a counterbalancing effect from my meals or supplements by afternoon. An adjustment in something so simple as having a well-lit, sunny workspace helped to turn this around. When I need more motivation, I sit in the sun or somewhere brightly coloured. Coffee can now be a treat, not a necessity.

# What Are You Doing Well?

When establishing our baseline, we are getting to know ourselves honestly that may go deeper than you are comfortable or familiar with.

We are our own biggest critics and often when we begin this evaluation process we forget to take a moment to view the things we deserve praise for.

Knowing the areas which you are currently doing well will not only build confidence but will help you to tailor a program which is really well suited to your strengths and which plays on this to achieve best results.

So let's begin, what are you currently doing really well?

For example, maybe you recognise that you don't yet have the ideal diet, we'll come to that shortly, but perhaps you consistently drink 2-3L of water. Perhaps you remember to take your multivitamin each morning. Maybe you're an excellent sleeper and always make sure you get your 7-8 hours bed rest no matter what.

Maybe you exercise several times per week, or perhaps you just never miss Monday night yoga.

Whatever it is, take a moment to write down the things that you are currently doing to take care of yourself. We can use this as a foundation to build a solid platform for change.

# What Are Your Skills?

Now that we've identified what you are already doing well and evaluated your starting point, it is time to take a moment to recognise your skills, strengths and weaknesses. There may be some that can be practised, enhanced, worked on and built. There may be some that require assistance from others. There will be some that are the cornerstone, the foundation of that bold and beautiful you - let's get to know these right here and now.

Ask yourself, what are you most proud of? Are you kind, nurturing and generous? Maybe you're bold, brave and a natural leader? Perhaps you're neat, organised, tidy and always on time, or maybe, like me, you're a little messy, quick-witted, often late but great in a crisis and great at thinking on your feet.

If you're suffering low self-esteem, then this task may seem overwhelming. Ask some of your loved ones for help if you're struggling. Ask the person who you trust most what they think your strengths are. Recognising your strengths can be the most powerful way to improve your self-worth.

Knowing your strengths also helps you to understand the best way to move forward with any change and can help to get better results from any life-change. Let me give you an example:

Though I'm very good at thinking on my feet and great at living in the moment, I'm not great at planning large projects. Unlike most people, I've never had a business plan, I've never been able to make projections, I find the whole thing far too stressful. I'm likely to jump directly into a project which I believe is a good idea. If it turns out well then great. If it fails I rarely get too stressed, I just move on or will adapt and change, this can lead to some lost time and money, but each experience is a lesson learned.

I decided to use my ability to adapt quickly to my advantage and, for more natural and authentic talks and workshops I now rarely script them. I choose the topic, research the idea and put a slideshow of interesting facts together. Then I just get up there and do it. This results in a fun and natural experience that is very much a conversation between me and the audience.

This has also been great for combatting stage-fright. I used to get incredibly nervous before public speaking engagements, mostly because I was going against my strengths and was trying to script, plan, write and learn a speech ahead of time. I then spent 1-2 weeks prior not sleeping, anxious that I would forget my talk or that it would not be good enough. I'd rewrite and rewrite in my head over and over (often in bed at night when I should be sleeping).

Now I speak to the crowd, not at them. It is a much more fulfilling interaction. Many attendees have told me that they find me more natural, authentic and engaging than other speakers which is always lovely to hear. Maybe it's because I now am having a conversation with them, enjoying the experience of being there with them, gauging my talk on the interaction with the crowd and adapting according to the response I am getting and what they need.

As a result of this change, I no longer feel stressed, I look forward to the event and leave feeling proud and confident that I did the very best

I could. I've gone from someone who used to give public talks for free to build my business (while secretly dreading it and being wracked with anxiety) to now being paid as a health speaker and thoroughly enjoying and looking forward to each engagement. I leave now feeling happy, fulfilled and buzzing with excitement, rather than thinking "thank goodness that's over" or "that was terrible, I should have done better".

Knowing my strengths is all well and good, but I also need to recognise my weaknesses to succeed as a business owner. Knowing I'm not good with planning and preparation, I took courses, paid for coaching and mentors and, where needed, I delegated the work to others who were better at it than me. I also learned from my mistakes of course, and yes I made plenty.

An excellent example of where failing to plan worked against me is with my internship. I set this up with all good intentions after being contacted by a Nutrition student in need. I had mentored practitioners for many years in my previous job managing a health clinic and remembered my own insecurities when starting out, so I understood her needs and felt ready to help. Shortly after we had an opportunity to take on more students. I came up with a way that they could get the industry experience they needed while helping me to run my business more smoothly. I did need some extra help at the time, so this seemed like a win-win. I took on an additional four students and, with the bare minimum of planning, welcomed them into my practice.

The first 6-9 months of my internship program taught me the most about my strengths and weaknesses as a practitioner. The chaos that ensued by not having planned, coupled with my innate nature of putting others before myself had me burned out and dreading going to work each day. My mother came to visit Australia and stayed with me for 3 months. I was stressed and working the whole time. I barely ever had a free minute to spend just relaxing with her, and when I did it, I was filled with guilt over neglecting her rather than enjoying the time we spent.

Ultimately something had to change. I picked up the leftover pieces of myself and, with some help from others, figured out what was working well and what was not working at all. I have refined this program until it put the needs of my patients first. All of my interns now are thoroughly briefed about the fact that they are there to work, that the patients come first, and that for the patients to get what they need from me, my needs also need to come a very close second. As a result, they now get an honest and practical experience of what it will take to run their own successful practice. They experience the hard work, the determination, the ups and the downs. If they make mistakes, they correct them! No more me running around after them leaving me feeling exhausted, depleted, and unable to coach or mentor them effectively. Ultimately I had to become more organised, more effective and less willing to put the minute by minute needs and demands of others before my own.

Not only has this transformation helped me to be a better practitioner and mentor, but the experience I had with my internship has also taught me a lot that I aim to carry through into motherhood. Selflessness is a good trait, but it is unsustainable in the long term. You have to take care of yourself, you cannot give from an empty cup! I gave, and I gave until there was nothing left of me during those early days. I was an ineffective mentor, too stressed and busy to provide them with any real coaching and too busy because I was shielding them from the actual work, correcting their mistakes, and never putting my own needs first. How could they possibly learn how to be a competent practitioner if they didn't know any of the hard work that went into it?

I now use what I learned there to help stressed-out mums to find their health and happiness again. I can speak from real experience when I say that real health and happiness and effective mentoring (what motherhood really is in a nutshell) cannot be achieved without giving yourself the love and respect you deserve.

# What Do You Need Most Help With?

So now that we've identified some areas which you're doing great in, it's time, to be honest about the areas you need the most help. These are the areas that need the most attention, the areas which maybe you know you need to change, perhaps you even attempt from time to time, but you just can't seem to break through and make it stick.

While we are our greatest critics, and we can see what we are doing wrong, often it is tough to admit we need the help of others to achieve the necessary changes. If you have been hurt, abused, neglected or lied to, then it can be hard to trust people, and yet this is sometimes when we need the help most.

An inability to know when to ask for help and an "I can do it myself" attitude is something I often see in my practice and is indeed something I have struggled with terribly (and often unknowingly) over the years.

Often I'll have people coming to me who have been trying to lose weight for 5-10 years or even more, before asking the help of a Nutritionist. Their health may be progressively declining, their weight creeping up despite several attempts - indicating that the approach they are taking is not working, yet still, they try to do it alone.

My stubborn and independent attitude comes from my upbringing.

From a young age, I learned that independence is the most reliable pillar of strength. I hid my feelings and attempted to be strong and put on a brave face for others - until I reached my breaking point.

From what I've observed in my patients, most of us tend to do this. Only the very secure and confident, those who have grown up in stable, loving, secure homes seem to be comfortable asking for help. However, even happy, healthy, stable adults can lose this confidence if in asking for help they are let down.

## Asking for help

I think the biggest revelation for me has been to understand that life is a team sport and that our team functions better when we know and work with each other's strengths and weaknesses. We have to expose and know them to be able to do this. You get the best help when you're comfortable sharing your shortcomings as confidently as your strengths.

The thing about team sports is that every player counts. Even the players on the opposite team have an effect on your performance! You are all playing together, even when you are playing against each other.

If you were watching a game of basketball, netball or any sport really, you'd get frustrated watching that one player who just won't take the help. How crazy would it be to see one "team member" trying to hog the ball, refuse to pass and still expect to get every winning shot? We wouldn't see them as a hardworking, downtrodden player. We would see them as one who is letting the whole team down.

There are times in life where you do have no one other than yourself to count on. There are things that you'll need to do alone. Just don't come to think of this as your only option and try to ask for, and accept, help when you need it. Many of the happiest, most successful people in life admit that they would not be where they are today if it was not for the help of others. I know I couldn't have written this book were it not for the support of my partner, the encouragement of my friends, and the dedication and expertise of my editor.

For me, this was my biggest hurdle in finding true health and happiness as a consequence of my experiences during my youth. Of course, every set-back, pain or negative experience as an adult initially then confirmed and solidified my feelings that I could only count on myself. This led to me pushing people away at times when I needed them most. Sitting alone in the dark rejecting phone calls from others who would happily be there when I needed it. Ultimately this also has led to lots of bad decisions over the years including accepting an abusive relationship as normal because no one knew about it to be able to tell me any different.

When you stop thinking of your life as a solo sprint and start participating in the team sport that it is, you may initially feel vulnerable. However, in reality, you will be putting yourself in a position to thrive, and you'll open up the opportunity for others to shine too. You'll allow others to express their real talent and the gratification of helping you. There is nothing better than helping someone who is in need. Sometimes there is no greater need than the help, love and support of others.

In short, when we recognise where we need the most help and reach out for it, not only do we lift our burden and give ourselves the opportunity to progress, we also allow others the joy of being part of the process, the pleasure of being useful, valued and needed.

# Setting SMART Goals

SMART goals are achievable goals. SMART goals are:

S: Specific, to ensure focus
M: Measurable, to ensure you are progressing
A: Agreed upon, to assure you are accountable
R: Realistic, to ensure you are capable of success
T: Time-based: in this case, 1 week each

Use this principle to map out some goals for each week of this program that will be achievable. It may also be helpful to set yourself some general goals for the program.

What would you like your life to be like in week 8? How do you want to feel? What would your new normal look like?

Use the SMART goals acronym to ensure that your intentions are specific, measurable, agreed upon, realistic and time-based. Doing so will significantly improve your ability to succeed.

## Why we need SMART goals

Picture this. It's New Year's Eve someone asks you "What's your new year's resolution?". You reply that you would like to lose weight / quit smoking/exercise more etc.

Because you haven't set yourself SMART goals your intentions may be short-lived. You start well, take advantage of one of those January gym deals paying very little for the first month or two. This is perfect, you think, as you can get into it before paying out. You head to the gym a few times in the first week, it is hard, but it feels good. You realise you do not have enough gym clothes, you go and buy some new pieces. You sleep better, eat better, feel better.

Then comes the first day you skip the gym, you have to work through lunch. Never mind, you will pick it up after work... except you don't. You stay back at work far too late and then wake up tired, grumpy, too late to head in before work. You grab breakfast on the go, usually something that doesn't quite meet the standards of what you'd make yourself at home. You tell yourself you're doing so well and you deserve a little break.

Now it's been a week, still no gym, you are tired, you have worked late most nights, you are not sleeping well, and your coffee intake has doubled, you are feeling more stressed and anxious throughout the day and are craving bad foods. You don't want to admit it or recognise it just yet, but your new healthy habit is broken. You may not exercise consistently again for some time. The more time that passes, the larger and more exhausting the task seems. You've lost your mojo.

## SMART goals help to maintain motivation

This is a story that I see all too often in my practice. Every January I'm working harder than anyone I know, with busy overbooked days and back to back patients all eager for change. Here I really stress the importance of SMART goals - if we aim too high, don't have accountability, or simply make unrealistic goals we're likely to fail.

While we all have great motivation in the beginning of a new venture, life often gets in the way and motivation is flipped towards powering through the life demands. Health-focus slips as we lose ourselves to long days in the office trying to get on top of that never-ending to-do list, chasing success, recognition and fulfillment. I know how it feels, I was there myself a while back.

While I was studying Nutrition, I managed a health care centre and for a while also worked at a detox clinic in my spare time. I loved my work. I ran both places like they were my own. I poured my heart and soul. Those clinics received more nurturing and care than my own body.

When I finished studying I got promoted in one of my roles, which quickly began taking over my life, largely due to my own choices. The more successful I became in my role, the more my health-regime slipped. I'd stay back at work until 9 pm in one workplace as, after 6, when everyone left I could finally get stuff done. No distractions, more satisfaction. I'd tell myself I was happy staying back and that I was doing it because I want to, that it wasn't stressing me, that I was calm and relaxed there and that this was no different to relaxing in front of the TV, only more satisfying.

I was becoming very "2 dimensional" - work, sleep, work, sleep, work, sleep etc. I loved my job so much that I forgot to take time out to take care of my friendships, I rarely took time out for my family. I rarely exercised unless it was walking to and from or a quick yoga session at work, all while still studying full time. I was burning myself out all over again. No amount of gratitude from my employers or colleagues would counterbalance the physiological consequences of the stress I was putting on myself.

## Setting SMART goals to achieve your goals

In 2014 I decided to make the giant leap to working for myself after 5 long years. I knew that staying in my current position meant I'd never do more than seeing a few patients on the side while giving my heart (and health) to the needs of the clinic. Walking away was a tough decision. I gave up a guaranteed income, I gave up control of roles that I loved so much and gave up many of my beloved patients.

However, this was the best decision I've ever made. Now I own 2 successful businesses, I run them with the values that are dear to me and work the hours I choose. In early 2015 I kick-started an industry-first internship program for students and new graduates of Nutrition and Dietetics (which I love) and last year I achieved a life-long goal of working as a volunteer health worker in a 3rd world country. I am giving my all to building a life I love. I wouldn't change it for the world and wouldn't reverse my decision to go it alone if I was offered tens of millions of dollars.

Of course, it was not all roses from the beginning. My first year out on my own was hard. I struggled without a steady income and the enormity of the work ahead of me to build my future was often overwhelming. To combat this, I set myself daily, weekly and monthly SMART goals and, though it took a while to see the fruits of my labour, in the end it payed off.

Now my work-life is balanced, my health is excellent, I'm happy and fulfilled, and with a baby on the way, I am lucky enough to be able to earn an income in my PJs if I choose. But none of this I could have achieved if I hadn't have been honest with myself, or allowed myself to get lost in the enormity of all that needed to be done.

If you're currently in a similar situation where work, or other demands, are taking over your life, and you often find yourself losing sight of what's most important to you then make sure you start setting SMART goals today and be sure to maintain this approach throughout the program. I want you to get as much out of our time together as possible.

Maybe today you start by setting a goal of reading a few chapters this week or of finding one change and committing to it. Don't let anything get in the way of your health. Setting SMART goals each week can help to maintain optimum focus and motivation throughout the busiest and most stressful of times, and can help to ensure that you continue to prioritise your health.

# Baseline Questionnaire

N ow that you've read a little more about the key points which make up your unique self, let's take time to complete the questionnaire below to set you up for a successful 8 Weeks. Use your answers from the questionnaire below to formulate your SMART goals.

## What is your starting point?

1. What does healthy mean to you? For example, are there any symptoms of ill health which you'd like to be free of in order to feel healthy and happy?
2. What areas of your self-care are you currently doing well with?
3. What areas of your self-care program might you need some help with? Who might be good support to help you with this?
4. What do you find usually gets in the way in the early stages of achieving your goals? For example: I run out of time to make my own meals/might have to work late and eat at my desk. Write down these factors now so that you can be prepared - be brutally honest.
5. What can you do to get around these roadblocks? For example: I will prepare a plan for the week and pre-cook my weekly portions of lunch and dinner on Sunday.
6. What factors would positively affect your motivation and energy? For example: emotional support/seeing or feeling certain changes/ having clear goals etc.

7. What factors do you think would positively influence your ability to relax?

So now you have taken my quiz, you understand a little more about where you are beginning. Now I want you to really think about where you'd like to end up. What does healthy mean to you? What does it look like? Feel like? What are the benefits you are feeling from this new found healthier, happier lifestyle?

Will you be playing a sport? Will you feel energy to burn? Will you be running along the water each Sunday morning with a smile on your face?

Will you be waking feeling rested? Will you sleep deeply? Will you feel calm, cool, clear and focused for most of your day?

Will you crave healthy foods and experience no sugar cravings?

Will you be drinking less? Will you be able to get through whole weeks with no end of day wine or end of week cocktail now that you are calmer, happier, more in control of your emotions?

Will you, my friend, look in the mirror and see a body you like? Will you feel comfortable shopping for clothes knowing that you'll find a range of options in most shops which suit you?

When you've had some time to consider these thoughts, write down some bullet-points that resonate with you. From here we can begin the really fun part which is tailor making a step-by-step plan to help you reach those goals in the next 8 weeks, and to maintain them in the years that follow.

# What Healthy Means To Me

# III

# Week 1: Simple dietary changes

# What Is a Healthy Diet?

Ahealthy diet is one which is nourishing and health promoting. It is a diet that leaves you energised and inspired at mealtimes. You should be looking forward to your meals and know that each meal will leave you feeling healthier than you did prior. You should never feel overfull/tired/ in pain/ bloated; portion control is an instrumental part of your healthy diet.

Your healthy diet will differ from mine, from your partners, from your friends'. We are each unique and therefore so must be our diet. However, there are some fundamentals and foundations that our individual intake must be built upon to preserve optimum health and well-being.

Your healthy diet should provide all essential nutrients through the course of a day. You should have adequate serves of vegetables, healthy fats, protein and healthy carbohydrates. Indulgences and treats should also be as healthy as possible, and you should not be relying on any quick highs from sugar or caffeine.

This week we're going to focus more on how to eat, rather than what to eat. However first let's have an overview of what to (and not to) eat this week. Focus on how you can improve each meal and snack. Small daily changes will add up, leading to a healthier, happier you without feeling overwhelmed.

So let's consider the ideal day, then we can work backwards from there.

## Getting the day started

Your breakfast is your opportunity to replenish after a night of healing, detoxifying and growing, mentally and/or physically. You will wake depleted of many vital nutrients and will be dehydrated. The quicker we refuel with valuable nutrients and water, the faster we fire up ready for a successful day.

Your digestive system really needs a lot of water to do its job, so we should begin by replenishing water. A 300ml glass of water 20 minutes before your breakfast can do wonders for your energy and can assist with naturally reducing coffee cravings and the urge to over-eat. In his book, *The Miracle Morning* author Hal Elrod discusses having a glass of water next to your bed and drinking it immediately when you wake up.[1]

Hal is right, rehydrating is the quickest way to wake up and actually the reason we sometimes feel tired when we wake up is purely dehydration. Correcting this quickly can lead to better energy and motivation which makes it easier to make healthy food and lifestyle choices. Adding lemon juice to the water assists the liver to recover from a night of detoxing and also further enhances your hydration due to the naturally contained electrolytes (minerals which control fluid absorption).

Now that we've rehydrated it's time to begin replenishing the nutrients needed for a successful, energised, healthy and happy morning. There are 3 key ingredients which are essential for all main

---

[1]  The Miracle Morning By Hal Elrod. https://www.miraclemorning.com/

meals, including breakfast.

## Protein

Protein helps with building and maintaining essential structures in our body which keeps us healthy. It also assists with regulating mood, hormones, blood sugar and sleep. We'll discuss protein in more detail next week, for now, let's focus on where to find it.

You should eat protein with every meal, but don't worry you don't have to eat meat for breakfast. Protein is found in varying amounts in all foods including meats, fish, eggs, dairy, nuts, seeds, legumes, and smaller numbers in whole-grains and vegetables. I often see protein to be the key feature lacking in a healthy breakfast, which leads to mid-morning energy slumps and increased cravings.

Consider now if you have protein in your morning breakfast and ways that you could upgrade the meal and add a little more.

## For example:

- If you currently eat cereal: You could add raw nuts, seeds and/or natural unflavoured yoghurt.
- If you currently have toast with butter and/or jam: You could switch to a natural nut butter such as almond butter and then sprinkle with a few more seeds, could switch butter and jam for ricotta with a little honey, or could top with a dense protein source such as eggs and avocado or sardines with lemon juice.
- If you currently have oats: You could add some raw nuts and seeds, could cook oats with water and mix egg through while heating (this is surprisingly good), could reduce the serve of oats and add

in some ground flax seed meal, or could top with some natural yoghurt.

## Ultimate Breakfasts:

Tip: You'll find the below breakfasts in the recipe section at the end of this book.

- Veggie-packed omelette - great for mornings with time for a hearty homemade breakfast.
- Homemade granola - delicious all year round. Can make single serve as needed in just a couple of minutes, or prepare in advance to sail through a busy morning.
- Homemade Paleo Banana Bread - delicious, ridiculously healthy and easy to make in advance for a healthy morning breakfast or mid-morning snack.
- Flourless choc-banana pancake - when you want a guilt-free indulgence.
- Protein Packed Super Smoothie - For blitz and go mornings.

## Carbohydrates

Healthy carbohydrates are a vital component of each meal and are essential for maintaining life. We get carbohydrates from almost all foods, other than meat, fish and eggs.

While it is possible to obtain healthy carbohydrates from healthy foods such as fruits, vegetables, nuts, legumes and seeds, us busy people often tend to revert to the starchy carbohydrates, such as potato, white rice, bread and pasta. While these foods are okay to include as part of a healthy, balanced diet, they shouldn't be the staple, as they are relatively low in nutrients in comparison to many other sources.

I would recommend limiting your intake of bread to just 1 serve of 2 slices per day maximum.  This leaves an allowance for the morning toast, lunchtime sandwich or bread with soup on occasion, but is restrictive enough to encourage that we increase other healthy carbohydrate sources such as fruits, vegetables, legumes, nuts and whole, unrefined grains.

Consider now how you could modify and improve your carbohydrate sources.

## Here are some examples:

- If you currently have a sandwich for lunch, you could try switching to a salad or wrap containing vegetables or salad with protein source of meat, fish or legumes.
- If you currently have toast for breakfast, you could try switching to whole rolled oats, homemade granola or any of the "Ultimate Breakfasts" listed above.
- If you currently have white rice with dinner, you could switch to quinoa, brown rice or even lentils. Another option is cauliflower rice, but we'll get to that shortly.
- If you currently have potato with dinner, you could switch to pumpkin, sweet potato or a larger serve of other vegetables.
- If you currently have pasta or noodles with lunch or dinner, you could try switching to spiralised vegetables such as Zoodles (zucchini -noodles).

## Healthy Fats

There are healthy fats and unhealthy fats. We will come to discuss this more next week, however, for now, let's just clarify that fats are indeed essential and therefore necessary as part of a healthy diet.

The types of healthy fats which we need more of are found in fish, raw nuts and seeds, avocado, olives, organic eggs, extra virgin olive oil, coconuts and coconut oil.

Consider now how you can improve your intake of healthy fats. Here are some examples:

- Dress salads with extra virgin olive oil, flaxseed oil or macadamia oil and/or include fresh avocado and olives.
- Add coconut oil, coconut yoghurt or coconut milk to smoothies.
- Replace 2-3 serves of meat per week with an oily fish such as sardines, salmon, mackerel or trout.
- Snack on raw nuts, half an avocado dressed with lemon juice or a veggie sticks dipped in nut butter or hummus.

## Fresh Fruits and Vegetables

We need a minimum of 6 handfuls of fresh vegetables each day and should enjoy 2 to 3 serves of fresh fruits.

It is important to eat seasonally and to buy organic where possible. If you do not buy organic, wash your fruits and vegetables in a mix of 1tsp baking soda, 3tbsp lemon juice and water to remove pesticides while preserving nutrients. The skins of fruits and vegetables are the most nutritious but are also where the pesticides are concentrated. Buying organic helps to reduce the nutrients lost through pesticides, peeling and scrubbing.

## Tips for eating more vegetables

- Eat your greens: green veggies offer the highest level of nutrients per calorie meaning you can eat tonnes of them, even if you are trying to lose weight, without blowing your "calorie budget." However, all colours are important and offer significant benefits, and most vegetables are relatively low in calories.

- Eat vegetables as snacks: Don't underestimate the power, or enjoyment, of eating veggie sticks with hummus or celery dipped in almond butter. My patients, friends and colleagues will tell you I am known for being seen around Sydney with a bag of raw green beans in hand, snacking on them as others do potato chips. Green beans, snow peas, carrot sticks or celery are also my go-to snack at the movies (sneaking them in of course).

- Drink Your Veggies: Juices are good for a quick vitamin & mineral boost, as the lack of fibre allows rapid absorption. However, the lack of fibre also creates a faster release of sugar. If you are trying to lose weight, balance your blood sugar, or are battling chronic thrush or systemic candida, you are likely to benefit more from vegetable and fruit smoothies.

- Juices vs Smoothies: With a juice we have removed the fibre to create a thin liquid. In a smoothie we simply blend the whole food with water. In a smoothie, you have broken many of the protein and fibre bonds that slow the release of nutrients, yet the fibre is still present to delay the release of sugar. I recommend putting vegetables in every smoothie, even if this means just a handful of rocket or baby spinach to your banana, yoghurt and berry breakfast smoothie. Sneak in a serve of veggies whenever you get the chance.

- Replace starchy carbohydrate sources with vegetable substitutes: Try lettuce leaves to wrap your burritos. Try spiralised zucchini or carrots in place of noodles. Try stir-fried grated cauliflower in place of rice. Try mashed cauliflower and zucchini in place of mashed potato.

When you eat this way, you should feel naturally energised and satisfied from your meals. You should rarely have the urge to deviate from your new diet because it offers everything you need and yet is still delicious and varied enough to keep it interesting. There will be times when you need to treat yourself just for the sake of it; I'll be providing lots of ideas of healthy indulgences throughout this program to assist with curbing the craving while staying on track.

# Is Your Diet Healthy?

I cannot tell you the number of times I've heard the patients in my practice who are struggling to lose weight, battling chronic digestive issues, candida, acne, depression etc. say "I have a really healthy diet". However, further analysis identifies many areas in need of improvement.

Maybe they eat the occasional salad for lunch, and for this, they feel quite virtuous. However, they are also eating cereal for breakfast, drinking too much coffee, eating fast foods or junk food "occasionally" (usually more often than they realise) and giving in to sugar cravings after almost every meal.

With a thorough review, we are able to determine the components of the daily diet which need to be restructured, removed or replaced for better health and happiness.

The following chapters aim to provide you with deeper insight into developing a healthy base-line diet. From there, we'll build each week by incorporating further therapeutic foods and continuously reassessing for additional modifications which may be beneficial.

# Creating a Healthy & Sustainable Diet

Taking time for the eating experience can help us to reduce cravings, control our portion sizes, and optimise our digestion - leading to higher nutrient yield from every mouthful.

This week we'll discuss the 5 foundations of a healthy sustainable diet:

1. Eating more fruits and vegetables
2. Portion control for optimal health
3. What to do when eating out
4. Optimising digestion through healthy habits
5. De-stressing meal times for better enzyme release

These are the factors which I'd like you to really focus on this week. Let's establish some great foundations and a healthy attitude towards food as medicine.

# Eat More Fruits & Vegetables

To support optimum health, energy and well-being your diet must be rich in fresh fruits and vegetables, with non-starchy veggies taking pole position. A diet rich in fresh fruits and vegetables helps to preserve a healthy digestive system, promotes healthy elimination of toxins, protects the kidneys from damage, maintains a healthy balance of gut bacteria (more on this later) and provide many essential nutrients required for repair.

Ideally, we want a minimum of 6 handfuls of fresh vegetables, and 2 serves of fresh fruits per day. For those who want to take it a step further, the following guidelines will assist you to make sure your vegetable intake is even more therapeutic:

- **Eat low GI:** Low GI, non-starchy vegetables should make up 75-80% of your intake. Most veggies are low GI, those that aren't include potatoes and beetroot.
- **Eat raw:** where possible, and appropriate eat your vegetables raw or lightly cooked such as steamed, steam-fried or stir-fried. These methods preserve the beneficial antioxidants, vitamins and minerals. Note: stir-frying is only healthy when a good quality oil such as olive, coconut or macadamia is used.
- **Eat fermented vegetables:** these are the front runners here and offer not only the vitamin and mineral boost but also are an excellent natural source of probiotics (good bacteria). The fermentation process also means the nutrients are more easily absorbed. Examples of commonly used (and widely available)

fermented veggies are sauerkraut, kimchi and pickled cucumbers. Top tip: fermented vegetables are our only food source of GABA (gamma-Aminobutyric acid) our primary anti-stress mechanism for switching off panic attacks.

- **Eat 6 handfuls of vegetables each day:** Aim to make this your minimum, if you can eat more than 6 handfuls then even better. Doing so can increase your energy and boost your mood in a matter of days (it's scientifically proven).[2]

A note about the starchy and sugary vegetables: Starchy and sugary vegetables such as sweet potato, pumpkin, potato and carrots are still a very healthy choice and should be used as the bulk of your carbohydrate intake most days rather than rice, pasta or noodles.

These vegetables offer nutrients such as beta-carotene, which helps to detox heavy metals from the body, and resistant starch which helps feed good bacteria in the gut. Starchy vegetables are a much more nutrient dense source of carbohydrates than most grains and are far superior to processed grain products such as pasta or white rice. Enjoy these vegetables as a side dish to your main meals.

## Eating Vegetables - The Insurance Policy

Increasing your vegetable intake offers an incredible number of health benefits. Studies show that increasing veggies in our diet results in:

- Easier weight loss

---

[2]  References

1. *Evolution of Well-Being and Happiness Increases After Increases in Consumption of Fruit and Vegetables.* **A, Mujcic R J Oswald.** 2016, American journal of public health, pp. vol: 106 (8) pp: 1504-10.

2. *Let them eat fruit! The effect of fruit and vegetable consumption on psychological well-being in young adults: A randomized controlled trial.* **M, Conner T Brookie K Carr A Mainvil L Vissers.** [ed.] van Wouwe J. 2017, PLOS ONE, Vol. vol: 12 (2) pp: e0171206.

- Improved kidney health
- Improved digestion and elimination (easier pooing)
- Improved control over body temperature
- Improved mood and mental wellbeing
- Enhanced detoxification
- A healthy appetite and reduced cravings
- Improved energy
- Improved exercise tolerance
- Enhanced healing response.

With a list such as this, I believe we can summarise to say that they can be seen as an insurance policy and a way to safeguard your health, improve your energy and to counterbalance many of the stresses of daily life.

Let's consult with 21-year-old Jen for a moment. 21-year-old Jen is unhappy, she's tired all the time, and no amount of sleep is helping.

We know she's also staying up all night on weekends drinking too much, abusing her body in an attempt to escape her emotions and her unfulfilling life. We know she's in an unsafe home environment, yet she's too worn out to do anything about it.

Now let me tell you something amazing. If Jen was to increase her intake of fresh fruits and vegetables, studies show that she'd feel happier, healthier and more energetic in days. Now that's worth a shot, right?

But here's the incredible thing. If Jen was to eat a high volume of fresh fruits and veggies every day, not only would she feel happier and more energetic, she'd also improve her general outlook on life. Her strength (physical and emotional) could improve, and she may just realise that she is worth so much more than this awful, stressful life that she is currently living. She may just have the resolve to pack her bags and leave - before this situation got really really threatening.

Unfortunately, 21-year-old Jen did no such thing. She continued to eat to survive, rather than thrive. Continued to drag herself through each day. It would take a while before she came to her senses. But we'll get back to this later.

# Portion Control for Optimal Health

What you eat is most important, there's no doubt about that. However, it is possible to over-eat even healthy foods and cause digestive distress, fatigue and weight gain.

I wish I could deny this fact. I wish I could tell you that as long as you eat healthy foods, it is almost impossible to gain weight - I really do, I know lots of others will argue that until they are blue in the face. But unfortunately, this is not true. Calories do matter, not as much as nutrients mind you, but they do count, and therefore we must be mindful.

Eating a healthy, perfectly portioned meal which suits our body's specific needs, means that we get the optimum balance of nutrients, without overloading on calories or stressing our digestive system.

So how do we figure out how much we should eat? To demonstrate how crazy our typical portion sizes are, I would like you to do an experiment for me. Place your 2 closed fists together side by side, with the palms facing each other and fingers touching. This is roughly the size of your stomach.

From looking at this, doesn't it make some of our regular meals seem excessive? Consider that pizza that you eat each Friday night, the rice or noodle dish you eat more frequently than you'd like to admit. Could they fit comfortably in this space? Is there any room for vegetables on top?

## Why we shouldn't overeat

When food begins to fill the stomach and the lining stretches, stretch receptors activate and signal a feeling of fullness. If we regularly eat more than our stomach can comfortably fit, our stretch receptors will be less responsive, and it'll take more and more food for us to feel full.

The little circular muscle that shuts off our oesophagus (the tube which carries food to the stomach, a highly alkaline, sensitive tube), from the stomach, may also weaken in response to overeating. This can lead to acid reflux, indigestion and heartburn, as acid sneaks through and burns the highly sensitive tissue of the oesophagus.

## What is the ideal portion size?

A general practice among Nutritional Medicine practitioners is to recommend using your hands to measure out your ideal portion size. This is an effective method in most cases as your hand size usually increases in synchronicity with your frame size, and therefore your nutritional needs. A large male for example, with a large hand and frame size will have higher requirements than a small female with small hand and frame size.

Personally, I like this method also as it is much more universal and practical than having to estimate cups, grams or tablespoons. We may not always have a measuring jug, but we always have our hands.
- **Protein:** Consume a minimum of a palm-sized portion of protein with each meal. If fish or vegetarian protein choose the size of your full hand.
- **Carbohydrates:** Consume a serving of carbohydrates no larger than your closed fist. If you're not currently exercising, skip the

carbs in some meals for improved results.

- **Vegetables:** Consume 3 handfuls of vegetables with each meal.
- **Fats:** Consume at least a thumb-sized serving of healthy oils with each meal. This would be equal to about a half tablespoon of olive oil or avocado.
- **Nuts and Seeds:** Consume a portion of nuts and/or seeds that is equal to what you could balance on 3 fingers.

An alternative is to measure a medium plate, around 30cm, no larger. Fill half the plate with veggies, no more than 1/4 the plate with carbohydrates and 1/4 of the plate with protein. While this is not quite as personalised as the hand-measuring method, this is still a good way of making sure you achieve a healthy balance within each meal. See the following image for a review and example.

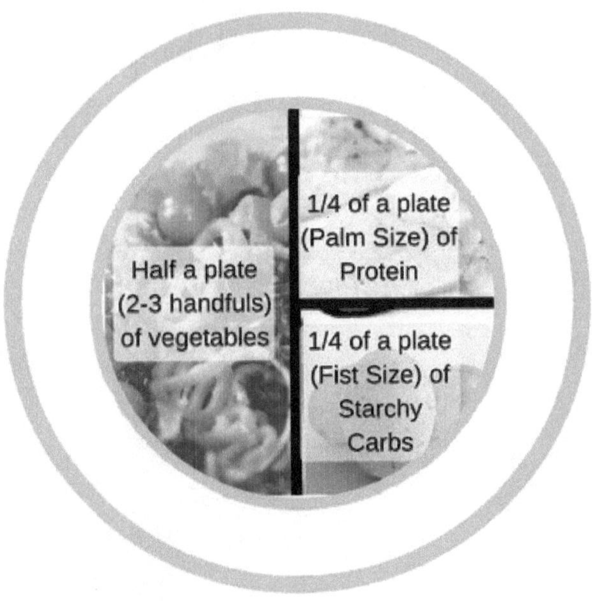

Now let's consider the size of your stomach again.  How does this meal appear to fit? Wouldn't you agree that this is a better balance? It allows you to get sufficient protein, fats, vegetables and carbohydrates without overstretching or straining your stomach wall.  This leads to appropriate signalling that you are full, better satisfaction from your meals, improved ability to digest foods and better absorption of nutrients.

# Eating Out Without Giving Up

Eating out - The modern twist on an ancient practice

We are social beings and sharing food is a practice which dates back several thousand years. There are many instances where we enjoy eating for pleasure and community building. This can be an excellent way to connect.

Historically, eating was almost always a fun, nurturing and very social event, often even celebratory. Food was shared among families or even villages, and we saw mealtimes as social collaboration.

There are many cultures where communities continue to eat together. I saw this in my time volunteering in Myanmar, where many in the rural villages still practice community eating. Pregnant women and children were prioritised, and people would often have smaller portions to make allowance for those in need.

In the western world, we still have this practice with a modern twist, where this urge for the social, community style eating, can be observed in the cafe culture. In many cosmopolitan cities, we consider it normal to enjoy eating out at restaurants and cafes several times per week.

So, if this is the modern day replacement, why is it that in cultures that still promote community eating, we observe healthier eating practices and lower rates of illness and obesity. Yet in cafe-culture societies such as Australia and America, we see obesity rates as high as 1 in 2?

Humans, like all animals, love to feast and enjoy putting together a feast for our loved ones. When we eat more than we need we often feel privileged, wealthy and successful (even if just for a moment or two).

When we practised real community eating, there was a collective interest in providing healthy, nourishing meals that would sustain the community for longer periods of time and to promote the health of each individual. We would also eat only what we need, as greediness could lead to others going hungry.

By contrast, restaurants have a financial gain from our indulgence. They have a vested interest in making us eat more than we need and to make their foods addictive (by adding excess cream, sugar and/or salt) so that we want to go back again and again. When you recognise this, you can make a choice – eat out less, or just make healthier choices.

Consider the following two scenarios:

1. A grandmother and mother cook for a large family event. They care deeply about each person attending and take measures to ensure that the needs of each are met.  The family members attending are mindful that there is a finite amount of food available to feed all. Anyone who overeats reduces the available food for the other family members.
2. A chef cooks for a restaurant of hungry patrons. The ingredients have been provided by the restaurant owner, there is more than enough to go around.  If the patrons eat more than they need the restaurant makes a higher profit, no one (except maybe the staff) goes hungry. In fact, the more money the restaurant makes, the more successful the chef becomes. Staff are encouraged to

provide dessert menus, to encourage side dishes, you are invited to eat as much as possible.

Considering this information, it comes as no surprise that eating out frequently can make it difficult to stick to a healthier diet. However, this is part of our culture, and it is time that we face it and put measures in place to allow us to enjoy this experience without the need to compromise on our health goals. Eating out can easily be incorporated into a healthy lifestyle plan, as can feasting, we just need to do it right.

## How to enjoy a healthy balanced diet when eating out.

## Tip 1: Read the menu in advance.

Most cafes and restaurants now offer a digital version of their menu online. When making plans, it helps to pre-read the menu so that you know your choices in advance. This is particularly important if you have any special dietary restrictions such as gluten free, dairy free or vegetarian.

By reading the menu in advance, you can take time to choose the healthiest option, or even ask your Nutritionist for assistance in selecting the best option for you and your health goals. You also have time to find out if the restaurant is open to menu item modifications. Would they allow you to swap the chips for a healthier side such as steamed vegetables, salad or new potatoes?

## Tip 2: Research restaurants with healthy menus

Do your research and find restaurants that have healthy menus and healthy desserts.  Follow some local health practitioners, fitness fanatics and even local celebs on social media.  This is one of the best ways to stay "in the know" about where to eat.

The rise of the healthy restaurant is prolific, particularly in major cities. However, you may be surprised where these are found. Ask your Nutritionist, personal trainer or local health food store clerk where they eat. There are new and exciting places opening up all the time.

## Tip 3: Tell your friends

I would really encourage you to advise those you'll be eating with that you are currently making an effort to eat healthier foods.  By doing so, you will be given the opportunity to brainstorm restaurants and cafes that will have a wider variety of healthy foods on offer. Not only will this make it easier for you to stay on track, but it will also enrich the experience for all involved. This also gives your companions an opportunity to be supportive, and to consider if they would like to join you in your efforts.

You'll be surprised how many people are relieved and often excited to have a buddy who will encourage them to make healthier choices. After all, we're never short of negative influences pushing us towards unhealthy foods.

As a rule, I generally avoid restaurants that don't have any healthy options on offer. However, if the situation is out of my control, I may eat a healthy meal beforehand and then just have something small, or I'll choose a couple of side dishes.

This is not to say that I never enjoy an unhealthy indulgence, of course I do.  However I only do so very occasionally and by choice rather than necessity. I am rarely stuck making the best of a bad lot. This helps me to maintain a gluten-free, pescatarian, healthy diet while still enjoying a fulfilling and active social life.

# Optimising Digestion

Digestion begins in the mouth where we secrete enzymes such as salivary amylase (in saliva) which helps to break down food. Improving digestion begins with the smallest and most obvious of steps - chewing your food.

## Take Time to Chew

If we do not take time to chew correctly (ideally until the food forms a paste) we are unlikely to digest our foods properly. This may lead to poor nutrient absorption (leading to deficiencies, poor food choices, sugar cravings, energy slump etc.), indigestion and fatigue.

With every morsel of food, we are saying to ourselves, "I choose to live". However with our current, rushed, unappreciated eating experience, we are missing out on this valuable component of the eating process. This means that we also miss out on the dopamine rush which typically results from consuming food. Our body recognises this lack of dopamine and, as a result, tells us to eat something which is an express path to dopamine release, typically chocolate or anything sweet.

Chewing your food and taking time to enjoy the experience of eating, also assists us to enjoy the sensual experience of food, without the need for unhealthy foods or overeating. We can get great enjoyment out of very healthy foods and smaller portions as our experience, and digestion is greatly enhanced.

## Don't drink with your meals

When we drink liquid with our meals, two things happen:
1. Firstly we are diluting our stomach acid - a vital enzyme which helps to break down protein and separate essential nutrients from their fibre bonds. Without adequate stomach acid we can become protein, iron, zinc and B12 deficient, and suffer from bloating, gas, constipation etc. due to inadequate digestion.
2. Secondly, when we drink with our meals, it's all the easier to swallow large morsels of food without chewing.

If you must drink fluid at meal times, aim to make it no more than 100ml. The end goal should be that you hydrate well throughout the day and take meal-times off to focus on eating.

## Don't rush your meals

When we chew our foods, not only to we taste the food and signal the release of stomach acid, we also send signals to release pancreatic enzymes and bile. The more time we take to chew and enjoy our meals, the more information our taste receptors pick up, resulting in releasing exactly what we need to digest and absorb our crucial nutrients from food.

When we rush our meals we cannot digest them properly. There simply isn't time to absorb or recognise enough information to trigger the release of appropriate enzymes, bile and stomach acid. As a result, we feel bloated and uncomfortable, occasionally also with reflux. On a deeper level, we are in more trouble, as inadequate digestion leads to deficiencies of nutrients which are essential for maintaining life.

It would be impossible to achieve pure health and happiness while suffering with nutritional deficiencies. Our moods, motivation, health and energy are intimately linked to the nutrients we eat. We'll discuss this more in future chapters and throughout this program. I'm sure, as you gain a deeper understanding, you'll come to wonder at the power of nutrition and the marvel of our bodies.

## Why is digestion important

Your digestive system is really your most important system of organs. This system takes on the daily vital role of absorbing essential nutrients to maintain your life. Without crucial nutrients, many of our organs and tissues fail. Malnutrition does not just come from a lack of food. Malnutrition can also result from a dysfunctional digestive system (or of course poor eating habits).

Throughout this program we will be working on many factors which optimise your digestive function, from improving sleep, separating drinks from your meals, eating healthy balanced portions and reducing stress. We'll also be discussing food intolerances and other conditions which inhibit digestion.

The better your digestive system functions, the more nutrients you absorb. Ultimately this leads to getting more out of each meal and allows you to fill up and meet your nutrient demands from smaller portions, leaving you feeling fresh and energised, rather than stuffed and bloated.

Later in this program, we'll discuss therapeutic foods which enhance digestion and how to further optimise your diet to support the health and function of your digestive system.

For now, stop washing your hurried mouthfuls of food down with big gulps of water. Take time to enjoy your meal, chew thoroughly and swallow without the need for a drink of water. In return, you'll find you crave fewer sweets, feel full for longer, and naturally adjust to healthier portion sizes very quickly as your hunger is reduced. You should also notice that you feel less bloated and gassy after eating and experience better digestion and more comfortable bowel movements.

**Tip:** It also takes a little extra concentration to properly chew your food, which provides a calming, mindful practice that can also reduce stress. We will come to the practice of Meditative Eating, and also discuss the digestive process in greater detail, in later weeks.

# De-stress Your Mealtimes

If you are eating on the run, in front of the TV, in front of a computer while doing work, or even on the phone checking emails, messages and social media, you are not focusing on your food. This leads to poor digestion (we'll get into the details of this later), can lead to overeating and often means less enjoyment of foods (which leads to craving sugary treats after the meal).

Take time out to enjoy your meal and create an environment for relaxed, unstressed eating, and you'll notice a significant improvement in your ability to maintain a healthy diet. If you focus on your food, taking time to see it, smell it, taste it and chew it, really enjoying the experience of eating, then everything, even a green leafy salad, becomes a flavour filled delight which you can look forward to.

This week I'd like you to take time out to really focus on enjoying your meals. This often means planning in advance to have enough time to do so. Plan adequate time to sit, relax, breathe deeply, appreciate the meal in front of you.

A good tip is to sit with your meal, close your eyes and take a few deep breaths. Enjoy the environment around you. Whether that is the sun on your face, a refreshing cool breeze or even the joy of eating in your favourite spot, your home or the most beautiful part of your office, appreciate these pleasures.

When you begin to eat, do so slowly, appreciate the smells, the colours, the flavours and the textures. In short, eat like the French. Enjoy the sensual experience of eating.

It is often helpful to also practice gratitude for the meal. You could choose to feel grateful for the fact that someone made the meal for you, that you are fortunate enough to be able to afford food, or for the ability to create your own meals. Appreciate that few minutes where you are choosing to nourish your body. Every time you put that fork, filled with healthy, nutritious foods, to your lips, you are telling yourself that you love and appreciate yourself, that you deserve good health and that you deserve to feel fabulous.

If you feel yourself rushing, getting distracted or losing focus, take a breath and remind yourself silently "Don't miss this" simple, yet powerful words for improved mindful living.

# Week 1 Summary

In Week 1 We Are Making a Commitment To:

De-stress our meal times and take time to relax and enjoy our food for optimum absorption and digestion.

When eating out, we are going to prepare by choosing healthy options in advance and choose appropriate portion sizes which will assist in further reducing the stress surrounding meal times. Also, we are going to take time to chew and enjoy our meals, reducing stress and healing the relationship with food.

We are going to eat more fresh fruits and vegetables, meaning we can fill up on healing, healthy foods which nourish our body and lift our energy and well-being in a matter of days, while also helping us to stay on track with our health and happiness goals in the long term.

We are going to eat appropriate portion sizes, which we eat mindfully and chew thoroughly. We will make sure that our plate is perfectly balanced.

Finally, if we eat out, we'll take the time to research the places in which we can enjoy the experience of social eating, while also maintaining our healthy diet.

# Week 1 Reflection

By the end of week 1, you should be enjoying your mealtimes a little more. Healthy eating should have become an enjoyable experience that is calming, restorative and nourishing in many ways. We should be enjoying better energy and feel happier and more positive, thanks to a healthy intake of fresh fruits and vegetables.

This is your foundation week, from which we will build. There are many more ways that we can enhance your diet to make it more personalised and more therapeutic of course. This will come. However, for now, I hope you're enjoying the transition, have become more conscious with your choices and are feeling that this change is practical, enjoyable and sustainable.

Now it's time to reflect on what we've learned and experienced in our first week.

Ask yourself the following questions.

- What did you learn this week that created the most significant change in your diet and/or mindset?
- How will the lessons learned this week change your life moving forward?
- What were you most excited to learn?
- What, if anything, were you most shocked or disappointed to learn?

# IV

# Week 2: Supercharge your diet

# Eat a Rainbow of Colours (Candy not included)

Last week we discussed the true meaning of a healthy diet and incorporated many practices to improve our daily intake of essential nutrients. This week we're going to build on this foundation by incorporating some therapeutic foods for greater health and happiness. Let's begin with the importance of "eating the rainbow".

Many people eat a diet which is mostly white, cream or brown. While there are healthy foods that are naturally this colour (such as garlic, cauliflower, mushrooms and potato) if we stick to the same colours our diets will be lacking in vital vitamins, minerals, anti-aging antioxidants and other incredible plant compounds.

Each colour in nature represents an entirely different nutritional profile. Each new colour, therefore, offers a new and exciting opportunity to improve your health. A healthy diet must contain a diverse mix of colours.

Make an effort to include as many brightly coloured foods as possible including red, orange, yellow, green, and purple, to ensure that you get enough of the essential plant compounds that have incredible and life-changing health benefits.

Each time you prepare a meal, consider how you can add an additional colour to the plate. Each individual colour represents unique nutritional properties (and therefore unique healing powers).

Why is each colour so important? That's simple, the colour is largely due to the "phytonutrients" they contain. Phyto = Plant, Nutrient = Vitamins, Minerals, Antioxidants etc.

Studies consistently show that people who eat more plant-based foods are healthier and happier and have a reduced risk of chronic diseases such as heart disease, diabetes and cancer. What's more, a study of more than 12,000 people, conducted by the University of Queensland, found that those who increased their intake of fresh fruits and vegetables felt healthier, happier and held a more positive outlook on life in general after just days.[3] From my personal and clinical experience, I'd say that this is intensified when we also ensure to consume a variety of colours.

------

[3] References

1. *Evolution of Well-Being and Happiness Increases After Increases in Consumption of Fruit and Vegetables.* **A, Mujcic R J Oswald.** 2016, American journal of public health, pp. vol: 106 (8) pp: 1504-10.

2. *Let them eat fruit! The effect of fruit and vegetable consumption on psychological well-being in young adults: A randomized controlled trial.* **M, Conner T Brookie K Carr A Mainvil L Vissers.** [ed.] van Wouwe J. 2017, PLOS ONE, Vol. vol: 12 (2) pp: e0171206.

# Why The Rainbow? The Health Benefits Explained.

Naturally Red Fruits and Vegetables:

The plant-based compounds found in red fruits and vegetables help to protect and repair our bodies from damage at a cellular level. Many of these compounds are said to reduce inflammation, boost immunity, protect cells from damage, improve heart function and protect from major diseases including cancer.

The most famous compound in red vegetables is Lycopene, one of the most potent antioxidants discovered to date.  Lycopene has been studied for a range of health benefits from preventing cancer to reversing macular degeneration.

After suffering a tumour that caused me to lose my vision temporarily, I upped my Lycopene and now make sure to consume a fair share every day by snacking on cherry tomatoes, red apples and cherries, adding raspberries and beetroot to my smoothies and packing my salads with tomatoes, radish, beetroot, pomegranate and red peppers. This is also important given that I have a family history of cancer. It's such a simple modification to my daily diet and yet has powerful protective effects.

## Naturally Orange Fruits and Vegetables:

Orange foods protect the skin, eyes, cardiovascular system and, again are instrumental in defending (or recovering from) cancer.

There are many valuable plant compounds in Fruits and Vegetables which assist in promoting health. Compounds such as Betacarotene, Bioflavonoids, Curcuminoids and Alpha-carotene, are responsible for the orange colour in foods such as carrots, pumpkin, sweet potato, turmeric, mango, papaya, oranges and apricots. These compounds are antibacterial, anticancer, antioxidant and anti-inflammatory.

The health benefits include better immunity, clearer skin, improved vision and eye health (Bugs Bunny had it right after all), cancer prevention or improved recovery and improved fertility. I'm always mindful to let all my pregnant (or trying-to-get-pregnant) ladies know to eat lots of orange foods. The betacarotene in orange foods also helps to detox heavy metals out of our body, and converts to vitamin A for healthy skin. So if you have a lot of mercury fillings, or you suffer from eczema or acne, these are the foods for you.

Easy ways to increase your intake of therapeutic orange foods include snacking on carrots, add turmeric to cooked meals and mix with olive oil and lemon juice for a healthy dressing, include pumpkin and sweet potato in main meals or make a healthy pumpkin soup to snack on. Swap summer icecreams for blended frozen mango and swap your bottled sweet salad dressing for blended mango and fresh lime. Snack on Papaya, oranges or mandarins between meals.

## Naturally Yellow and Green Fruits and Vegetables:

Yellow foods contain healthy plant compounds such as Lutein (think eye-health), Rutin (think healthy arteries) and Zeaxanthin (which protects your macula which is responsible for vision). Green foods contain a long, long list of plant compounds including chlorophyll (think of this as plant-blood, a highly nutritious compound), Folic acid (for healthy babies and protection from cancer), Indole-3-Carbinol (for healthy hormones) and Sylimarin (think healthy liver) among many, many others.

Like the orange foods, yellow foods are anti-cancer, anti-inflammatory and help to promote eye, skin, cardiovascular system and also the brain. Green foods are the real superfoods, containing a plethora of health-boosting compounds which are anti-cancer, anti-inflammatory, antioxidant, detoxifying, hormone regulating, and protect almost all organs and systems in the body from damage.

The health benefits of eating more green vegetables include reduced inflammation and easier healing from injury. Higher exercise tolerance plus quicker and more efficient recovery. Improved immunity, clearer skin, healthy balanced hormones, improved fertility, easier weight loss, improved detoxification, reduced hangovers and of course cancer prevention.

Obviously, as a pregnant female, my greens are highly important. However we all want healthy hearts, reduced inflammation and more energy, right? I've seen drastic improvements in my patients' health when they've taken time to introduce more green and yellow foods. Dramatic improvements have been seen in many patients blood pressure and weight loss results.

- We can easily include more yellow and green foods by drinking water with fresh lemon or lime juice. Add mint if desired.
- Add a handful of spinach or rocket to your smoothies. Add frozen zucchini to your smoothie to make it thicker and creamier. Replace pasta with spiralised zucchini and serve with homemade pesto.

- Use fresh herbs mixed with extra virgin olive oil to create a delicious pesto which can be added to vegetable dishes, served with salad or add to spiralised vegetables.
- Snack on cucumbers, granny smith apples, green beans, celery or green peppers between meals. Blend spinach, lime juice, avocado and garlic to make a deliciously healthy dip for snacks or to serve with salads.
- Mash peas, zucchini and cauliflower with turmeric, garlic and co-conut cream for a delicious and healthy mashed potato substitute.
- Blend apple, mint, cucumber and baby spinach for a delicious, thirst quenching, anti-inflammatory, anti-cancer mid-morning snack in the form of a green smoothie.

## Naturally Blue and Purple Fruits and Vegetables:

Blue and purple fruits and vegetables are rich in nutrients which are, you've guessed it, anti-cancer, anti-inflammatory and protect the brain, heart and cardiovascular system (beginning to see a pattern yet?).

This food category contains some particularly delicious foods which, in my opinion, get used far too infrequently. Blue and purple foods are a great way to boost the appeal, flavour and texture of your meals while also increasing your intake of many essential nutrients.

In the blue and purple foods, we find plant compounds such as resveratrol (think anti-aging and better blood sugar control), anthocyanidins (anti-oxidants) and hydroxystillbenes (improved memory and sharper brain function).

Health benefits of blue and purple foods include healthier eyes and improved vision, healthy liver and improved detoxification, improved cancer prevention, improved focus and memory and controlled blood sugar for a healthy appetite and reduced cravings.

A study by the University of Cincinnati found blueberries improved memory, focus and learning ability in elderly adults with dementia after just 12 weeks. This is a great representation of the power that Nutritional Medicine holds. [4] While these studies were looking at reversing dementia and alzheimers, we can all apply these findings to help reverse the damage caused by stress (which often mimics early signs of these conditions).

We can include more blue and purple foods by snacking on blueberries, figs, plums and prunes. Add grated purple cabbage to your salads and look out for purple carrots, purple kale and purple cauliflower too. Add figs to salads for a deliciously healthy nutrition boost plus a gorgeous contrast of flavours. Fig and cucumber salad with goats cheese, dressed in extra virgin olive oil is particularly delicious. Make vegetable lasagne and use purple eggplant strips in place of pasta sheets.

## Healthy indulgence alert

*Fancy a sweet treat? Why not add blueberries or acai berries to your smoothies or enjoy a snack of delicious fresh figs and blueberries with coconut yoghurt. Use blueberries as your natural sweetener when baking healthy treats or making home-made chocolate (see the recipes section for my homemade, dairy-free,*

---

[4] *Blueberry supplementation improves memory in older adults.* **al., Krikorian R Shidler M Nash T Kalt W Vinqvist-Tymchuk M et.** Cincinnati : Journal of agricultural and food chemistry, 2010.
   **https://www.ncbi.nlm.nih.gov/pmc/articles/PMC2850944/**

*sugar-free, blueberry chocolate bar recipe).*

## White and Brown Foods

White and brown foods are considered to be less nutritious as we generally associate them with polished white rice, white or brown bread etc. However, there are many naturally white and light brown foods which hold incredible benefits.  The problem with the afore mentioned foods is actually the way that they are processed, many of the nutrients have been removed.

Naturally white and brown foods provide many essential minerals and plant compounds which assist with liver function, boost immunity, support detoxification and improve digestive health. Examples of particularly beneficial white foods are cauliflower which enhances detoxification and can assist with balancing hormones, and garlic which is an excellent immune booster (garlic is antiviral, antibacterial and anti-fungal and helps lower blood pressure and cholesterol).

Healthy white and brown foods include cauliflower, potato, quinoa, chickpeas, brown lentils, mushrooms, raw nuts and seeds, raw cacao, coconut, brown rice, onions and garlic.  Black tea is also a highly therapeutic brown food.

## Food focus - Garlic

Garlic is an incredible white and brown food which holds significant healing benefits.  The benefits of garlic include; improved blood pressure control, reduced cholesterol, improved immune surveillance, improved white blood cell production. Garlic also can bring down a fever quickly and acts as a natural antibiotic, antiviral agent and is anti-inflammatory. You'll find a recipe for a garlic tea in the recipes section which I often recommend to my patients suffering from colds, viruses, or those with troubled immunity.

## Eating the rainbow for better energy

By increasing your consumption of colours, you will find your energy increases, and your overall health and happiness improve. This occurs for 2 reasons:

1. Firstly you will be exposing yourself to more of the beneficial and essential nutrients that each coloured vegetable and/or fruit has to offer.
2. Secondly, your meals will become more visually stimulating, and you will find that looking at your plate, filled with a wide variety of bright and vibrant colours, boosts your energy and appetite. You will find yourself craving more fresh fruits and vegetables and far less sugary or processed foods.

# Eating the Rainbow - Checklist

Top 5 tips for adding more colours to your daily diet:

1. Stock up on fresh fruits and vegetables - aim to fill your basket/trolley with as many brightly coloured fresh fruits and vegetables as possible.
2. At each meal, aim to include 3-4 natural colour varieties from a range of sources. When you're done and ready to serve, check the fridge and strive to add 1 more colour in the form of a dip, sauce or dressing.
3. Make smoothies by blending together fruits, vegetables and herbs. My favourite smoothies are baby spinach, lemon, mint and apple OR beetroot, blueberry, spinach and cacao.
4. Snack on brightly coloured raw vegetables such as; raw carrots, green beans, snow peas, sugar snap peas, chopped capsicum, chopped cabbage (purple is sweeter, green is juicier).
5. Dip chopped veggies in hummus, home-made pestos or nut butter. Try my homemade dairy-free "Super pesto" from the recipe section. I also recommend black bean hummus, beetroot dip and homemade cashew and coconut butter.

Review the checklists of foods of each colour over the following pages and use the tips above to incorporate more into each day. Set yourself a SMART goal for this week. A good goal may be to eat more of one colour food that your diet is currently lacking. Remember to keep the goal small, measurable, agreed upon, realistic and time based (I'd recommend a daily goal here).

This is a simple and very effective way to boost your overall intake of health-promoting vitamins, minerals and plant compounds without the need for any exotic super-foods or supplements. You'll feel the difference in a matter of days.

## Red Foods

Apples, Kidney beans, Beetroot, Blood Orange, Capsicum, Cranberries, Cherries,Chilli peppers, Grapefruit (ruby red), Goji berries, Grapes, Spanish Onion, Plums, Pomegranate, Potatoes, Radish, Raspberries, Strawberries, Rhubarb, Tomato, Watermelon

## Benefits

Anti-Cancer, Anti-inflammatory, Cell Protection, Gastrointestinal health, Cardiovascular health, Hormonal balance, Liver Health

## Ideas

Tomato, capsicum and onion salsa added to fish or chicken or enjoyed as a dip

Crushed tomatoes, capsicum, onion and chili for pasta sauces, soups etc.

Add Beetroot Pomegranate and Radish to salads

# Orange Foods

Apricots, Capsicum (Bell Peppers), Carrots, Mandarins, Mango, Nectarine, Orange, Papaya, Paw Paw, Persimmon, Pumpkin, Rockmelon (Canteloupe), Squash, Sweet Potato, Turmeric, Ginger.

# Benefits

Anti-Cancer, Anti-microbial, Immune Health, Anti-Inflammatory, Cell Protection, Reproductive Health, Eye Sight, Mental Health

# Ideas

Grate carrots through your salad or add capsicum. Mix up your salad by adding fruit such as mango, papaya or mandarin - these make great dressings.

Add carrots/sweet potato/pumpkin to pasta sauce

Drink Turmeric & Ginger tea (see recipes)

Use orange juice as a marinade for fish or chicken

## Yellow Foods

Asian Pears, Banana, Capsicum (Bell Peppers), Corn, Lemons, Millet, Pineapple, Summer Squash, Ginger

## Benefits

Anti-Cancer, Anti-microbial, Cell Protection, Memory & Cognition, Eye Health, Heart Health, Skin Health, Vascular Health

## Ideas

Dress salads with lemon or add to water or tea and enjoy as a beverage.

Drink ginger tea (see recipes)

Snack on bananas and pineapple.

Add capsicum and summer squash to your salads and stirfries.

91

## Green Foods

Apples, Artichoke, Asparagus, Avocado, Bean Sprouts, Bitter Melon, Buk Choy, Broccoli, Broccolini, Brussels Sprouts, Cabbage, Capsicum (Bell Pepper), Celery, Cucumber, Green Beans, Peas, Green Leaves & Herbs, Limes, Okra, Olives, Pears, Snow Peas, Soy Beans (Edamame), Zucchini (Corgette)

## Benefits

Anti-Cancer, Anti-Inflammatory, Cell Protection, Brain Health & Cognition, Heart Health, Hormonal Balance, Skin Health, Liver Health

## Ideas

Drink green juices and smoothies with a blend of green fruits and veggies.

Add lime juice & celery to avocado as a dip.

Add Broccoli, Zucchini, Cabbage, Green Beans and Green Leaves to omelettes, stirfries, salads.

Enjoy snacking on celery & cucumber.

## Purple Foods

Berries, Cabbage,  Purple Carrots, Cauliflower, Eggplant, Figs, Grapes, Olives, Plums, Potatoes, Prunes, Raisins, Purple Rice
Balsamic Vinegar (made from purple grapes)

## Benefits

Anti-Cancer, Anti-Microbial, Cell Protection, Brain Health & Cognition, Heart Health, Eye Health, Skin Health, Liver Health

## Ideas

Snack on Blueberries & Blackberries or make blueberry muffins/chocolate (see recipes).

Use Capsicum, Carrot, Cauliflower, Eggplant & Kale in Stirfries, Soups, Salads etc.

Snack on Plums, Prunes & Figs, or add to salads for a naturally sweet salad dressing.

Add balsamic vinegar to salads.

95

# White, Tan or Brown Foods

Apples, Beans, Cauliflower, Cocoa, Coconut, Coffee, Dates, Garlic, Ginger, Legumes, Mushrooms, Nuts, Oats, Onions, Pears, Sauerkraut, Seeds, Soy, Tahini, Tea, Wholegrains

## Benefits

Anti-Cancer, Anti-Microbial, Cell Protection, Gastrointestinal Health, Heart Health, Hormonal Health, Liver Health

## Ideas

Snack on Nuts and dates filled with tahini

Make healthy homemade treats from almond meal and cocoa

Add mushrooms to stirfries, omelettes and salads

Add beans, legumes and wholegrains to main meals.

97

# Digestion Boosting Foods

There are many foods which are fabulous for improving digestion. While some contain enzymes, others promote the release of acids, hormones and enzymes in our bodies. Including these therapeutic foods daily is the most effective, and cost-effective, way to improve your digestive health.

Below you will find a list of helpful foods. If you feel your digestive system could use some additional support, I would like you to choose 1-3 of these foods to include this week and to have those foods every day for a whole week. Ideally, I'd love you to have one or more at (or before) every meal, however, if this is unachievable simply pick the meal which you find you typically struggle most with digesting and use them then. For many people, due to the stress of work, this may be lunchtime, for others, it may be dinner.

These tricks I'm going to teach you over the next few weeks will support you for life, or at least as long as you continue to use them. They are invaluable, and I'm incredibly excited to share them with you.

You'll note that there are several foods to choose from, please select a food below which appeals to you most or which best fits in with your preferences. If you can implement several foods, this is even better, however, please aim to do this daily for the whole week.

## 20 minutes before eating

- Cup of strong green tea (note if you're iron deficient then you must not drink green tea within 1hour of eating as it can bind iron and reduce absorption)
- Cup of dandelion tea
- Cup of water with juice of half a lemon

## 5-10 minutes before eating

- 1 tablespoon of apple cider vinegar
- 1/2 a grapefruit
- 2 handfuls of rocket dressed in apple cider vinegar

## With a meal

- 2 handfuls of rocket / radicchio / bitter lettuce / dandelion greens
- 8-10 olives
- 1/4 cup of bitter melon
- 1/2 lemon juice / 1tbsp apple cider vinegar as marinade or dressing
- Coriander, dill, turmeric
- pineapple, apple, pomegranate and pawpaw

## After a meal

- Pineapple, Pawpaw, Papaya or Kiwi Fruit
- Apples - particularly when grated
- Lemon juice in water or strong green tea with lemon
- Half a grapefruit

# Protein

Protein is the essence of life. Protein contains amino acids, which are the building blocks for most structures in the body.

From protein sources, we get our "Essential Amino Acids" which are amino acids which cannot be produced in the human body and therefore must be consumed through food sources.

## Where do we get our protein?

Protein is found in almost every food source, with animal products such as meat, fish, eggs and dairy offering the highest concentration.

Vegetarian protein sources include beans, legumes (lentils, chickpeas, beans), tofu (made from soybeans), miso paste, nuts and seeds, nut and seed butter, green vegetables, especially broccoli and whole grains such as oats, quinoa and brown rice.

## Are all forms of protein equal?

All forms of animal protein contain all essential amino acids and are therefore referred to as complete protein. However most plant-based sources include some, but not all essential amino acids, therefore combining two sources assists in achieving the complete protein - think of rice and beans here. What the beans lack, the rice makes up and vice versa.

## How much protein do I need?

To calculate your specific protein requirements, multiply your weight in kgs by 0.8. This is the minimum number of grams of protein per day that you should be consuming to maintain muscle, energy and health in general. To make this easier, just eat 1 g per kg of body weight. So if you're 70 kgs eat 70 g of protein daily.

If you are quite sporty or are trying to gain muscle, then your protein requirements increase. Here you should multiply your weight in kilograms by 1 to 1.5. So for example, if you weigh 60 kgs, then you should be aiming to consume about 60-90g per day. This is easily achieved with a palm-sized serve of meat or fish at each main meal, some nuts or nut butter for snacks between meals, and eggs or a protein shake for breakfast. If you need an extra boost, a good quality protein shake blended with water or coconut water and berries can go a long way.

## Calculating your protein intake

To record or calculate your intake I typically recommend apps such as MyFitnessPal, EasyDietDiary or MyNetDiary. These will allow you to enter the 2 eggs you have for breakfast and will advise you that this equates to 12-14g of protein (depending on the size of the egg). Having this information allows you to tailor your intake to your unique needs and also teaches you how to make small adjustments to your regular meals for better daily protein.

# Healthy Fats

For decades media and medical reports had us thinking that fats were evil and we should eat more carbohydrates. Now we are told that fats are good and we should eat more fats, fewer carbs. Seemingly conflicting scientific discoveries have us spun into a frenzy. Do we go high fat low carb or high carb low fat? Both sides have very compelling arguments, who do we believe?

Let me just declare once and for all that fats do not make us fat! Excess calories, from any source, do. We have been trained to believe that by going low fat, fat-free or "skinny" that we can battle the bulge. However, if you look at the rates of obesity, they have climbed since we introduced higher carbohydrate, highly processed, lower fat foods.

Fats are a valuable and essential food group that are necessary as part of a healthy diet. Every cell in our body is wrapped in a fatty layer. We cannot live without them. The reason we became so fearful of fats is that we took a terribly simplistic view which seemed to make sense.

You see, fats contain 9 calories per gram, where protein and carbohydrates contain just 4 calories per gram. When you look at this with limited understanding, it's easy to think "then if I reduce my fats I reduce my calories". However, when reducing fats, you reduce your exposure to essential, fat-soluble nutrients which naturally reduce hunger, inflammation and cellular ageing, while also improving blood sugar control, mood, energy and hormonal balance.

Have you felt the difference that a tablespoon or two of avocado, a few nuts, some olives, feta cheese or even a creamy dressing can make to a salad? This is because fats are soothing, comforting and satisfying to humans. We are designed to love them because we need to ingest them in decent amounts daily.

## So what does this mean? Do we need to go low carb high fat?

The answer is no. All food groups are essential, and we merely need to make sure that we always make an effort to choose the healthiest possible sources and to get plenty of them. The most valuable lesson you can learn to improve your health is that every mouthful matters. You must make each and every forkful of food count. Choose the healthiest, most nutritious source of every food and you just cannot lose.

For a healthy, happy body we should fill up on healthy, natural, healing fats such as olives, raw nuts, seeds, avocado, oily fish and eggs. These fats carry essential nutrients which enrich our health, help us to control inflammation naturally, can reduce pain, hunger and fatigue, can enhance our mood and memory and improve our hormonal balance.

Unhealthy, processed fats, such as margarine, store-bought cookies, chocolate, chips, processed meats (such as bacon, prosciutto, salami, pastrami, deli sliced chicken, ham or turkey, sausages etc.) contain harmful, inflammatory fats which destroy our health from the inside out. These fatty foods increase our risk of heart disease and obesity and can worsen inflammatory disorders such as depression, arthritis, fatigue and fibromyalgia.

Fun fact: Some people have more of an affinity for fats than others and will often be found eating butter off the spoon, drinking cream from the carton, or requesting "extra crackling please" - yes I've done all of the above. I considered myself strange until I came across some interesting research.

It seems that certain blood types appear to require different amounts of fats in their diet. Blood type O, for example, actually seem to need a higher fat diet to maintain optimum mood and energy.[5] Without a decent serve of fats each day we are more likely to feel anxious, excessively hungry or even depressed. Blood type O's are those who will pour on the extra cream, oil and butter with delight where other blood types watch on in disgust. Even watching us can make them feel queasy.

Interestingly Blood Type O's also do better with endurance exercise (which burns more fat as fuel than carbohydrates), do not typically tolerate sugars particularly well (unless combined with fats to slow the release) and would be more likely to go for cheesy pastries, warm buttered bread or a creamy cake than a bowl of sugary sweets.

This is just one example of how fabulously individual we all are, and how just one diet rarely works for everyone. We are all unique and have our own unique needs and preferences. Our healthy diet should be as individual and unique as we are. For those who love fats, we can work with this. We can eat a diet rich in good, healthy fats and satisfy the body's natural cravings while simultaneously nourishing ourselves to the core.

---

[5]  "Eat Right For Your Blood Type" by Dr Peter J. D'Adamo

# Carbohydrates

Carbohydrates supply the body with the energy it needs to function. Found in most foods aside from meat, fish and eggs. They are the only fuel for our brain and blood cells and are the primary fuel for most others.

Carbohydrates are two groups – simple and complex - both of which are considered to be healthy when they are from natural sources.

Simple carbohydrates are sugars including sucrose which we know as table sugar, fructose which is the sugar naturally contained in fruits and vegetables, lactose (milk sugar) and many others. Fruit and honey are good examples of natural sources of simple carbohydrates.

Complex Carbohydrates are also made up of sugars, but the sugar molecules are strung together to form much longer, more complex chains which take longer for the body to metabolise. This is why we feel full and satisfied for longer after eating brown rice or lentils (complex carbs) than we do after equivalent carbohydrates from fruit or honey.

Complex carbohydrates include fibre and starches. Complex carbohydrates include vegetables, whole grains, legumes, nuts and seeds.

When we eat complex carbohydrates, such as grains, legumes, vegetables, nuts and seeds, we gain the nutritional benefits of the whole food, which typically results in higher energy, a healthy digestive system, balanced mood and controlled blood sugar.

An unhealthy subgroup of carbohydrates, which are the common cause of disease in the Western world are processed carbs. These carbohydrates, sometimes referred to as refined carbohydrates, are found in anything which contains white flour. Examples include pasta, white bread, pastries, cookies, some cereals and battered or crumbed foods.

We make white flour by removing the bran and germ from whole grains. The bran (rich in vitamins and minerals) and germ (rich in fats, antioxidants, vitamin E and B Vitamins) are the most nutritious parts of the grain. What we are left with in white flour is just carbs and proteins, without any of the nutrients that our body typically expects to receive alongside them. Eating these types of carbohydrates will lead to increased hunger and fatigue.

By consuming processed carbohydrates, rather than loading up on whole grains and legumes, we actually deplete our valuable nutrient stores and can end up creating deficiencies. For this reason, processed carbohydrates should be considered part of the occasional or treat food family, and should be limited in a healthy diet.

The typical western diet is too rich in refined, processed foods and too-low in fruit, protein and beneficial fats. This is detrimental to virtually all aspects of health and is known to cause:
- Insulin resistance, diabetes and obesity
- Increased appetite and sugar cravings
- Weight gain with poor metabolism
- Higher body fat and lower, poor quality muscle
- Accelerated ageing and skin conditions such as acne, eczema and dermatitis

- Higher rates of inflammation and pain
- Higher incidence of food intolerances
- Higher incidence of autoimmune diseases such as rheumatoid arthritis and Hashimoto's thyroiditis
- Record numbers of cancers and cardiovascular disease

This week I'd like you to review your carbohydrate intake. Could you modify your intake slightly? Where possible swap simple and refined carbohydrates for complex carbohydrates. Let's swap white rice for brown rice and/or lentils.  Let's exchange sugary, chemical filled sweet treats for fresh fruit.  Let's trade that white bread (including sourdough) for dark, grainy spelt or sorghum.

Trust me, you'll feel the difference.

# Sugar

Sugar is found in many natural, healthy foods in smaller amounts and is a safe, natural substance which our body knows exactly what to do with. Sugar is not an evil substance, nor is it something we must avoid. Very few people become unwell from eating naturally sugary foods such as carrots, apples or mangoes.

Recently there has been a tremendous amount of media attention on sugar, and rightly so. We needed to raise awareness for the added sugars that are sneaking in too many of our favourite foods for no good reason.

However, I'm finding that there is a lot of confusion about sugar, how much is safe and whether there are indeed safer sources. I find many people think that the highly processed rice malt syrup is a healthier option than organic honey, molasses or maple syrup, which is absolutely crazy.

Recently, when discussing the benefits of swapping the afternoon coffee with a small carrot and beetroot juice on one of my social media feeds, I had someone declare "But what about the sugar hit???" - Like I'd just told people to drink a glass of maple syrup. It's really getting out of control. We need to stop with the hype and come back to basics.

We've all been whipped into a frenzy, and no nutrition book would be complete without addressing this vital issue once and for all.

## So let's talk sugar!

### Is sugar evil?

Sugar is not evil, it is a necessary form of fuel. Only when we over-consume sugar in a pure or processed form does it become problematic. Natural sugars are not to be feared and should not be something you're putting too much focus on when trying to improve your diet. So yes you can continue eating fruit, sweet potato, carrots and corn woohoo!

### What are natural sugars?

Natural sugars are those which are naturally occurring in any particular food. For example, a carrot has 2.9g of natural sugars, an apple typically has 10g, a ripe banana usually has 12g, and 1 cup of chopped mango typically contains 23g of natural sugars. Who still thinks we need to be concerned about the "sugar hit" in a small, freshly made, carrot juice?

### What are added sugars?

Added sugars are those which have been added artificially during processing or cooking. They are there to enhance flavour and to act as a natural preservative. Most packaged foods contain higher amounts of added sugars to reduce the loss of taste during storage.

### Are any sugars evil?

There are some sugars which I feel we should be very fearful of and which do not have a place in a healthy diet. These are found in soft drinks, junk foods, flavoured yoghurts, pre-made sauces, marinades and dressings. These types of foods can contain vast amounts of added sugars from highly processed sources such as high fructose corn syrup. This is the type of sugar our body really has little evolutionary experience with and is not well equipped to metabolise. Often these products also contain sugar in far higher amounts than we would naturally consume by choice.

If you'd like to test this theory, I urge you to take your favourite soft drink or sweet treat and check the sugar content on the label. Divide this number by 4, and you have how many teaspoons of sugar this drink or food contains. Now take a glass of water and add the equivalent sugar amount. You probably won't be able to drink it without making yourself feel really sick.

The secret is that companies often add in high amounts of sugar which make the food highly addictive. Then they add in other substances to counterbalance the sugar and prevent nausea and vomiting. Unfortunately, however, these substances do not prevent the other health consequences which typically result both in the short and longer term.

I'd like you to consider this each time when reading labels from here forward. Try to choose lower sugar options whenever possible. If it's more than you could comfortably drink in your tea, then it's too much!

# Sustainable Changes

Now that we've learned the dietary principles upon which this program is based, it's time to consider how we make this approach sustainable.

It's all well and good to commit to a program, hoping to see a change and to be determined to stick with it no matter how hard. However what happens 6 months or a year from now, when you've forgotten how you felt in the beginning.

I don't just want to give you a program that helps you feel good for 8 weeks. I want to provide you with a program that allows you to develop healthy habits for life. We're aiming to work hard for 8 weeks yes, but this is just the beginning. (Unless of course, you are a fruit fly, in which case, if you make it to 8 Weeks, you are doing seriously, seriously well!)

So how do we make these changes sustainable? There are a few things to consider;

- **Choose the challenge less challenging to establish your healthy habits:** What do I mean by this? Well for example, if you hate zucchini then choosing this as your green vegetable and eating it 2-3 times per day is not really going to do you any favours. You'll suffer through every meal, and your suffering is unnecessary. There are plenty of other green veggies. Start with the ones you enjoy.

- **Make an effort with your meals:** Experiment with colours, flavours and textures. Try not to sit down to chicken and broccoli too often. You'll get bored, feel resentful and probably crave pizza.
- **Do your research:** Look for recipes that excite you. I've included some in this book to get you going, but this is only the beginning. The time you take to research healthy recipes will be paid back in full with that first bite of the "Oh my goodness, I can't believe I made this" meal.
- **Take your time:** Remember there is no rush here. Take your time, there's a reason I've called this an 8-week program rather than 8 days. It's important to go at your own pace, as long as you commit you'll see change.
- **Enjoy the process:** Our perception of health and happiness is very much relative. Enjoy the process of learning and empowering yourself with this new arsenal of self-discovery. Know that the more you put in, the more you get back but also be kind to yourself. There will be challenges along the way, and there will be tough weeks. Use your new found tools to get through this and these challenges will become a learning experience. Whatever you do, keep pushing forward. Every little effort counts.

Remember, when we begin to make changes, our body responds. If these are positive changes we usually get a positive response. This may happen very subtly; before you know it you feel better than you ever have before. However it is quite common to forget where you started. Now the expectation will be to feel this fabulous all the time... anything less is just plain unacceptable.

Be present through this process of change. Observe how much easier it is to face the challenges that present themselves if you continue to eat well and sleep well. You'll be able to see these challenges as a learning experience gifted to you to enhance your resolve. It is also helpful to journal your experience; note any challenges and how you got through them. There's a great web app for journaling called Penzu. For a physical journal, I recommend the Best Self Journal. Note any particular benefits you experience from your new found foods. This is all part of the journey to that healthier, happier you.

# Week 2 Reflection

This week we have expanded on our knowledge of how to build a therapeutic healthy diet. We've discussed the importance of each coloured fruit and vegetables, and have delved deeper into the important food groups.

Now it's time to check in.
- What resonated most with you this week? What are your necessary focus points?
- What SMART goals can you set for yourself? What do you feel is a comfortable first step, or one which you feel most passionate or excited about?
- What are your high priority changes? Do you need to modify your intake of healthy carbs, fats, protein and sugar, or do you simply need to eat a wider variety of colours?
- How will you set yourself up for sustainable change.

Next week we are going a little deeper into creating the ideal healthy diet by discussing some ways we can clean up our act with a low-tox diet.

# V

# Week 3: A low-tox diet

# Cleaning Up Your Diet

Last week we discussed ways that we can supercharge our diet with simple adjustments such as eating more colours, incorporating digestion-boosting foods and how to set ourselves up for more sustainable change.

This week it's time to look at cleaning things up a bit. We'll learn to optimise our health by reducing our exposure to unnecessary toxic burden and focusing on fresh, healthy, whole foods. This can have enormously beneficial effects on your mental well-being. In natural medicine we talk about the "angry liver"; whenever a person's liver is failing to keep up with their daily demand and toxins are accumulating, the person becomes angry, snappy, red-faced and unapproachable. If this is coupled with constipation, which it almost always is (as the same dietary mishaps cause each condition), then you have a swollen, snappy and scary human. There are a few reasons why this happens:

Firstly, to comprehend this, think of the liver like our personal assistant who is highly skilled and we could not live without. When the workload is manageable, things run smoothly. All daily duties are performed on time, the whole operation benefits. Now I'd like you to imagine that this same assistant has had more work to do each day than they can possibly get through (as with when we overload the liver with regular alcohol intake and unhealthy eating). The work is piling up and this assistant is tired, running behind and is slower than usual. However, the daily tasks keep coming, and they pile up on the desk.

Each time he/she completes 1 task, 5 more are added to the pile. Now it doesn't matter how many crucial and essential tasks are sitting on the to-do list, he/she simply cannot keep up with the work-load.

Clean eating takes away some of that stress and is like going over to that stressed out PA's desk and offering a helping hand. Taking away unnecessary tasks so that he/she can focus only on what's necessary. When we remove harmful chemicals, toxins and foods which make our body work harder, systems run better. The liver now can get through his daily to-do list easily and maybe with a little rest time to relax and recover.

Put simply, when the liver works well, all tasks it is in charge of get done on time. This includes digestion, removal of toxic wastes, hormonal balancing and many more.

Another reason is the impact of our digestive health on our neurotransmitter balance. We'll discuss neurotransmitters in greater detail later on. For now, let's just say that these are chemical messengers which control our mood. When well nourished, our body is capable of producing lots more serotonin (the happy hormone) 95% of which is produced in the gut, and only 5% in the brain. This is significant and could explain why we get so grumpy when we are clogged up.

The term "clean eating" is an alternative name for a gentle detox/cleanse. Put simply it means to eat a balanced diet, remove foods that make your body work harder and focus on healthy, whole food, fresh ingredients which provide essential nutrients.

This is an excellent way to initiate a gentle cleanse and remind your body (and your mind) of how great you feel when you eat wholesome, healthy foods. When we eat clean we eat more of the best and healthiest options in each of the food groups—and less of the not-so-healthy ones. That means embracing whole foods like vegetables, fruits and whole grains, plus healthy proteins and fats. It also means cutting back on refined grains, added sugars, salt and unhealthy fats.

Here are some helpful tips to get you started:

- Limit processed foods. Choose whole, natural foods instead -Many processed foods contain excess sodium, sugar, chemically restructured fats plus preservatives and additives which may deplete your valuable nutrients, beneficial bacteria and also disrupt the healing process. An easy way to clean up your diet is to look at the ingredient list on packaged foods. If the list is long or includes lots of ingredients that you can't pronounce, try to stay away from it. Better yet, avoid all packaged food. This is a tough one for some, but you will really notice the difference if you can do it.
- Increase your vegetables. Vegetables are full of vitamins and also high in heart-healthy fibre, which helps you feel full. Opt for dark green leafy vegetables which act as antioxidants in the body. Bitter veggies also actively improve digestion by increasing the production of digestive enzymes. We'll expand on digestive enzymes and foods which boost them further when we come to phase 2 of your recovery program in later weeks.
- Cut down on saturated fats. Your diet should be rich in good, healthy, anti-inflammatory, healing fats such as avocado, olives, olive oil, seeds, oily fish such as sardines, salmon or mackerel.
- Drink plenty of water. A dehydrated body functions less efficiently, delays or inhibits healing and causes you to crave unhealthy foods with salt and sugar. Your digestive system requires an abundance of water each day to function well. You can measure your level of hydration by looking at the colour of your urine, we'll discuss this further in later chapters.

# The Chemical Burden

In 2018 we are faced with more toxic chemicals than ever before. Our poor health has been blamed on everything from sugar to healthy grains and legumes. Foods like dairy and sugar have been demonised, and the recommended "healthy diet" has become a real shapeshifter.

Ask anyone you know why we are sicker in 2018 than ever before, and you'll no doubt receive many valid and arguable responses.

Across many theories, however, if you actually break them down, it comes back to the same, integral problem. The chemical burden.

Some examples are:
- The candida theory
- The gluten theory
- The food intolerance theory
- The sugar theory

I'll discuss these further over the next pages to keep you fully informed. For some, this may help to clear up some fears, fads and myths. For others, it may help with understanding why certain changes could be beneficial for you. If there's something which resonates with you over the next few chapters, feel free to incorporate it into your healthy eating plan. Otherwise, use this information to better understand what a healthy diet really is, and how it can be modified further for improved results.

# The Candida Theory

There is a type of yeast which lives in our system called candida. In healthy numbers, candida lives very harmoniously with our other microbes in the digestive tract and the vagina.

However, candida is an opportunistic microbe (meaning it will flourish and take over very quickly with the right conditions). When in high numbers, candida becomes parasitic, meaning it causes a decrease in health and wellbeing, draining our nutrient reserves and causing many unpleasant symptoms.

The health consequences of candida overgrowth may be something as simple as the discomfort of thrush which presents as burning, itching and production of white discharge in the oral cavity (oral thrush) or vagina (vaginal thrush). This is often seen after antibiotic use and with the use of steroid inhaler asthmatic medication (oral thrush).

Candida thrives in a high oestrogen environment and therefore may become a problem before menstruation and with the oral contraceptive pill.

Fungal skin and toenail infections, dandruff, cradle cap and athletes foot are other examples of chronic issues which may be caused by this microorganism.

More severe and debilitating conditions associated with chronic candidiasis are chronic fatigue, food intolerances and reduced immunity.

By minimising high sugar foods, and improving our tolerance of natural sugars, we can assist in the management of candida and prevent the troublesome overgrowth which is difficult (but not impossible) to reverse.

If you are suffering from chronic candida, chronic thrush, or any of the other conditions mentioned above, I urge you to see a practitioner of Nutritional Medicine. By changing your diet and supporting your body with natural medicines such as lavender, garlic, tea tree, coconut oil and clove, which are natural anti-fungal agents, you will beat this condition and be restored to full health in no time.

So where do the chemicals come in with candida? Where do I begin? Unfortunately, many of the chemicals which we are exposed to daily have hormonal altering effects. This causes imbalances which can lead to dysbiosis, can increase candida overgrowth, while also increasing our risk of many other major diseases.

The truth is our hormones are more out of balance than ever before, and in my opinion, it is due to the high exposure to tens of thousands of chemicals every day. These are chemicals which not only pose health risks, but unlike natural substances, our bodies are not equipped to deal with them, they don't even know what they are. We'll come to discuss this further in later weeks. For now, let's focus on optimising our diet.

# The Gluten Theory

As a life-long sufferer of gluten intolerances and owner of two healthcare businesses which specialise in the management of food intolerances, I can tell you that I am not entirely adverse to the idea that gluten is the root of ill health in many people. However, in most cases, the gluten is not the origin of the problem, it is merely the result. Seeing gluten as the root of the problem has led to misunderstanding and mismanagement, with many people continuing to suffer unnecessarily for many years.

With the rise of medical attention on food intolerance, we are treating them like most other diseases which is to avoid the trigger to reduce or prevent the symptom. However, I want you to use a little common sense for a moment for me. Something that many practitioners are not doing. If the body has become sensitive or intolerant to a food, yes it makes sense to remove it temporarily, but why aren't we asking why the sensitivity is there? If we don't find out what caused the reaction, then we may never find the cure.

Here's another analogy, food intolerances are the smoke, the symptoms (gas, bloating, fatigue etc.) are the smoke alarm. By cutting out the food, we are merely fanning away the smoke. This is not enough! To return to whole health, we naturally must find, and put out the fire!

## What is gluten?

Gluten is the collective name given to a group of proteins which are found in grains such as wheat, barley and rye, plus many others. To go "gluten-free" means to cut out these grains and their derivatives, therefore minimising your exposure to these proteins.

## Is a gluten-free diet healthy?

A naturally gluten-free diet can be a wonderfully healthy choice, when done well. Each swap can mean a significant upgrade to the nutritional balance of each meal. When going gluten free we can swap our sandwiches for salads, cereals for fresh fruit with nuts and seeds, a pasta dish for spiralised veggies with homemade sauce, and pizza for a homemade cauliflower pizza base topped with real ingredients. (You'll find many of these recipe ideas in the recipe section)

We also may swap processed treats for healthy homemade versions such as my quinoa flour chocolate cupcakes which are far more nutritious and can be enjoyed as a healthy indulgence guilt-free as they offer powerful, healing nutrients which actually enhance, rather than damage, our health.

However, the improvement here is not really down to the removal of gluten, the most significant improvement, in fact, is the introduction of more whole food ingredients, the increase in vegetables, and the reduction of processed foods.

## But wait, there's more...

For those who suffer from coeliac's disease or gluten intolerance, there is an even more significant improvement in their health by eliminating the exposure to gluten. However, while coeliacs disease is hereditary and, as far as we know to this day, irreversible, gluten intolerance is an entirely different story.

You see in coeliacs disease there is a genetic mutation which causes an auto-immune (the body attacking itself) reaction which is initiated after the person consumes gluten. It is an autoimmune condition, caused by a set of faulty genes, which is brought on by food allergy.

However, in gluten intolerance, there is a sensitivity, meaning the body has developed antibodies to attack the gluten protein every time it is consumed. This causes irritation, inflammation, toxic buildup and, due to an irritated, dysfunctional digestive system, nutritional deficiencies.

## What does it feel like to be gluten intolerant?

The symptoms of gluten intolerance are varied. Some people experience only digestive symptoms, some experience fatigue, depression, anxiety or weight gain. However, I must stress one more time that the food, the gluten, is not the problem. It is the body's tolerance of this food which has failed.

## Is gluten bad for humans?

In my opinion, gluten is not some toxic substance that no human should eat. Yes, it's true however that I personally eat very little gluten and do have to coach the majority of my patients by going gluten-free to restore their health. However, the gluten reaction is the result, not the cause. Yes, it is a result which leads to further complications. However, we need to look a little deeper to figure out the actual cause.

In fact, the cause comes down to chemical burden, no matter which way you look at it. There is an unknown number of possible reasons for gluten intolerance, and yet, all that is known to date can be attributed to the chemical burden. Here are a few examples:

## Cause 1: Dysbiosis

Dysbiosis is an imbalance of microbes (bacteria, yeasts, viruses) within our body and is the most common cause of gluten and other food intolerances. Dysbiosis is caused by stress, high sugar diet, low vegetable intake, nutrient deficiencies, restricted diet, anorexia nervosa, medications (especially the contraceptive pill, antibiotics and pain relievers) and hormonal imbalances.

However let's assume for a moment, that you're eating the perfect diet, consume only fruit sugars, do not take medications, are not stressed and have perfectly balanced hormones and nutrient levels. What is one thing that we cannot get away from in our environment these days? Well, that is unless you live in an actual bubble... CHEMICALS!

There are so many toxic chemicals that we are exposed to on a daily basis. If you could see the number your head may actually explode. We'll get into exactly where we are being exposed to the majority of our toxins later, however, for now, I'd like to teach you the hard and scary facts.

The United Nations Environmental Programme estimated that there are approximately 70,000 chemicals in regular use across the world. How scary is this?

Even more frightening is that these chemicals are often released without any prior testing or clearance required to demonstrate that they are safe and non-toxic! With 1,000 new chemicals being intro-duced every year, this is a genuinely frightening piece of information.

The National Institute of Occupational Safety and Health reported that nearly 900 chemicals used in cosmetics are toxic and that the estimate might be low.

So, before we jump ahead and summarise the chapter right here to say that all disease is caused by the chemical burden, let's come back for a moment to food intolerances.

I've mentioned above that dysbiosis is the primary cause of food intolerances. Well, what if I was to tell you that our little bugs, the good guys who maintain optimum health and balance in our system, are highly sensitive to chemicals. Our bodies are just not equipped to deal with them. Many of these chemicals are also known hormone disruptors, creating severe imbalances which have been linked to severe conditions such as endometriosis, infertility, birth defects and cancers. This is a highly detrimental state for us as humans and even more so to the microbes living inside our body, which of course control digestion, mood, metabolism, immunity, hormonal balance and the repair of many organs.

## Cause 2: Intestinal permeation

Intestinal permeation, commonly known as "leaky gut syndrome" is another known cause of food sensitivities. Here, the barrier in the intestines has been weakened, which leads to poor nutrient absorption (leading to deficiencies) and an ineffective filter system which no longer blocks absorption of food particles, bacteria, yeasts and viruses into the bloodstream.

As a result, there is a higher rate of infection, leading to the immune system being over-stimulated. When food particles enter the blood, your body recognises that this is a foreign body which should not be here, and tries to protect you by developing antibodies to "kill" or "attack". Each time you consume the food in question, these antibodies will aim to attack and defend you. However this heightens inflammation, may cause damage to structures within the body which have similar proteins and inhibits digestion and absorption of nutrients.

Cause 2 is often a direct result of cause 1: dysbiosis. Because these little microbes are in charge of the repair and maintenance of your digestive lining, when they are low, you are not sufficiently repairing. Couple this with an influx of harmful bacteria or yeast (such as candida – more on this next) and you have a digestive system which is under constant attack, with no "soldiers" to repair it.

Due to the required repair, you have a higher demand for nutrients, but your absorption is reduced. This is a vicious cycle of course as a damaged digestive lining does not absorb nutrients, and nutrient deficiencies mean you don't have the resources to be able to do the necessary repair.

Damage to the intestinal wall can be caused by dysbiosis, which we know can be caused by the toxic burden. However further damage to the intestinal wall may directly be caused by the chemicals themselves. Of the 7000 chemicals in circulation, remember most have not been tested or cleared as safe for human consumption when exposed to just one alone. There is certainly no data which can determine what may happen when we are exposed to a cocktail of these chemicals every day.

## Cause 3: Glyphosphate

Glyphosphate is a chemical compound used in the pesticide called "Round Up". The use of Glyphosphate appears to have increased at the same rate as Coeliacs disease and Gluten Intolerance. A fact which

Dr Stephanie Seneff, a senior research scientist at the Massachusetts Institute of Technology (MIT), found incredibly interesting and therefore has dedicated a significant period of time to research.[6]

Dr Seneff believes that Glyphosphate may be strongly correlated with the instance in coeliac disease and gluten intolerance, along with other severe conditions such as autism.

Glyphosphate increases the absorption of arsenic into the kidneys and aluminium into the brain. These toxic chemicals are incredibly damaging substances which cause an incredible amount of harm. The use of Glyphosphate in wheat agriculture is widespread.

Also, Glyphosphate, a pesticide designed to kill living things, is incredibly damaging to our microbes that control, manage, repair and restore our digestive systems. In effect, when we eat Glyphosphate treated wheat (which is all non-organic wheat), we might as well be taking a strong dose of antibiotics. We are wiping out vast colonies of our good bacteria.

As discussed in point 1, dysbiosis (bacterial imbalance) may cause food intolerances, leaky-gut-syndrome may cause food intolerances. Glyphosphate damages the lining due to chemical toxicity and depletes good bacteria which are both protective and in charge of repair of our intestinal barrier, making this a double hit to our digestive health.

As you can see, it's not the gluten that's the issue, its the chemicals which we are exposed to. Glyphosphate is just one of them, there are tens of thousands more chemicals which we are exposed to every day,

---

[6] S. Seneff, A.Samsel. Glyphosate, pathways to modern diseases IV: cancer and related pathologies. Journal of Biological Physics and Chemistry 15(3):121-159 · January 2015

many with dire health consequences.

# Food Intolerances & Elimination Diet

Now that we've established a few ground rules for what it means to have a healthy diet, some of you may have discovered that you'd benefit from taking it one step further. In the previous chapters we discussed candida overgrowth and gluten intolerance. Did either resonate with you?

If you are struggling from severe fatigue, chronic digestive upset (gas, bloating, diarrhoea, constipation) or chronic skin issues such as acne or eczema, and the changes you've made so far hasn't managed to improve this, then it may be time to individually tailor your diet to suit your specific needs.

You see, some foods will easily promote better health, better energy and will provide essential nutrients in a readily absorbable form. While other foods may be a little more challenging for your body to digest. If you are suffering from any food sensitivities, allergies or intolerances, these particular foods may be creating daily damage, irritating your digestive lining until it is no longer able to do its vital job of absorbing essential nutrients.

## The Elimination Diet

The elimination diet is a tried and tested way to determine your most therapeutic, and most damaging, foods. The idea is to cut out many foods which commonly cause reactions in many people for 3 weeks.

After this, you begin to rebuild your diet by slowly reintroducing the eliminated foods one at a time.

The traditional elimination diet is relatively strict, highly restrictive, and, in my opinion, often unnecessary as a first step. With my patients, I usually begin with a modified version of the elimination diet, starting by cutting out just 2 major food groups and then working from there. From what I've observed in my patients over the last 6 years, dairy and gluten-containing grains seem to be the biggest offenders. Therefore this is where we begin.

My 5 step approach, when working with someone who is suffering from fatigue, significant difficulty losing weight and/or digestive dysfunction is:

1. Correct the baseline nutrition: This means all the basics, improving hydration, increasing vegetable intake, reducing sugars and processed foods and ensuring adequate protein.

2. Introduce therapeutic foods and nutrients specific to the condition. For example, for people suffering from bloating, digestive pain, gas etc. I'd introduce probiotics, increase probiotic foods, introduce digestive enzyme boosting foods. For those suffering from persistent fatigue, I'd introduce energising foods, B Vitamins, Co Q10, Magnesium and utilise energising superfoods such as raw cacao, maca, acai berries and matcha.

3. Reassess, if the primary issue is not yet resolving, it's time to take it 1 step further. Here we'll begin the modified elimination diet. I'll guide the patient through how to remove gluten and dairy safely. We'll monitor any progress or improvements, and this will determine the appropriate next step.

4. If removing gluten and dairy has not resulted in adequate relief, it's time to begin eliminating other potentially problematic foods. Here we'll either perform a food intolerance test or start a full elimination diet.

5. Through the food intolerance test, elimination, or modified elimination diet we will have determined the foods which must be eliminated, those which should be reduced and those which can be eaten freely.

At this point, we now have a completely personalised diet. Here we can use appropriate therapeutic foods to improve overall health and wellbeing.

If there are food intolerances, then this means the digestive system needs to be supported and healed. I'll institute a 3month gut recovery program to restore optimal digestion and with the aim to be able to reintroduce many of these identified problem foods once completed. I teach my patients how to reintroduce foods safely and slowly, to find their tolerance level and to ensure they do not undo all the hard work done throughout the program.

If you have some lingering symptoms that you'd like to be free of and suspect you may have a food intolerance I'd recommend a 3 step approach.
- Step 1: Take what you've learned so far and modify your diet to be healthier overall.
- Step 2: Keep track of your primary symptoms/concerns (revisit week 1's questionnaire for a reminder) and monitor improve-ments.
- Step 3: If you are not yet experiencing improvements, or if you are feeling any worse, I'd recommend visiting a practitioner who can help you with a food intolerance test or elimination diet. Please don't try doing it alone, the elimination diet is very strict and restrictive and it is vital you receive the appropriate professional guidance to ensure that it is a safe choice for you.

Note: If you are diagnosed with food intolerances then, after your initial period of elimination we can rebuild you.  To find out more about the support available for sufferers of food intolerance head to https://www.foodintoleranceaustralia.com/support

# Should I "Quit Sugar"?

It wouldn't be appropriate to end this section without a discussion of going sugar-free, possibly the most popular (and the most excessive) dietary trend since the low-fat diet.

Firstly I must say that the "Quit Sugar" theory has been taken way out of context and becoming misunderstood, over-valued and over-discussed. In the process, many other essential factors are getting missed (or ignored).

I must mention here that when you "quit sugar", you initially may transition to a much healthier diet. It's not necessarily about the sugar, it's often about the fact that you're eating more healthy whole-foods which are not refined, processed or loaded with chemical toxins such as artificial flavours, colours, preservatives etc.

With the Quit Sugar diet being so difficult and often unsustainable, we should really ask the question: Do we really need to go sugar-free? Can we just eat healthier and achieve the same or even more significant health benefits?

We've talked previously about what sugar is, where it's found and the different types. You know that sugar is a natural substance found in many healthy foods, and can also come in the form of "Added Sugar".

## So why the hype?

Sugar is added to lots of foods. Many foods that are touted as healthy, such as bottled juices, flavoured yoghurts and salad dressings have added sugar, as sugar is actually an excellent natural preservative. Obviously, when we eat large doses of sugar, it is detrimental to our health as it causes large spikes, followed by dramatic crashes and, over time, may lead to a condition called insulin resistance where the cells no longer respond to the insulin released.

Why is insulin resistance a problem? Well you see we don't get energy from sugar, we make energy from sugar (and all foods) and this we do inside the cell. Now imagine this cell is a locked castle. Insulin is the "key" to the "lock" (insulin receptor), which opens up the "gate" (channel) so that sugar (glucose) can enter the cell and we can convert it into energy. Any sugar remaining in the blood after insulin release is considered to be excess and therefore converted to our 'back up storage reserves' which is body fat.

In the case of insulin resistance or type two diabetes, the "key" no longer opens up the "gates", so sugar can't get in (this means no energy and lots of perceived excess). So, in a nutshell, we become overweight and exhausted.

There appears to be a link between insulin resistance, obesity and cancer. Again another win for the Quit Sugar theory. However it's not the sugar that's the problem, it's how your body is handling it. Your body's response to sugar is largely determined by the form it comes in (what the total meal or snack contains or lacks).

Finally, because it is metabolised very quickly, sugar increases appetite. This appears to affect women more strongly. My theory is that this is a biological predisposition to assist us in our predated gatherer roles. If food was sweet, it was ripe and safe for eating, but not for long. We needed to be excited and stimulated by the sweet taste to enhance our ability to feast. Healthy men appear to be less stimulated by sugar and more stimulated by protein, which would make them better hunters. Again, this is just my theory, there are many others which may explain this occurrence.

On a physiological level, when sugar is consumed, we experience a rapid increase in blood sugar, followed by a significant insulin response, followed by a blood sugar decrease. Therefore it makes sense that we would be more hungry when eating sugar alone. However, sugar, when added to foods containing protein and fibre, such as in a salad dressing, can also result in mildly increased hunger. There is no blood sugar crash in this instance, and yet the result is similar. Our hunter-gatherer instincts perhaps?

So yes **excess** sugar consumption or a high intake of **processed foods with added sugar** may lead to many diseases. I'm very grateful to the Quit Sugar movement for raising the issue of **hidden sugars**. It has taken what we Nutritionists have been doing in our talks, blogs, newsletters, books and consults, to a global scale via cool articles, books and movies and now many people are sugar-aware. Even GPs who have long been known to dismiss the value of a healthy diet, have started discussing the impact of high sugar foods. I'm very grateful for that, it's helpful when we're all on the same page.

However, the demonisation of sugar, the encouraged restriction of fruits, and many other healthy foods is a step too far. And many people are missing out on well recognised therapeutic foods as a result.

## What about Rice Malt Syrup?

Another bugbear of mine is that the "sugar phobia" does not seem to extend to those sugars which are touted as healthy such as rice malt syrup. People are adding rice malt syrup to many recipes in place of fresh berries or bananas for example. A sugar syrup is always just a sugar syrup my friend. Yes, there are some which are worse than others, high fructose corn syrup, wheat syrup, these are evil sugars. However maple syrup, raw honey and molasses are, in my opinion, far healthier choices than the heavily processed rice malt syrup.

## A note on honey, maple syrup and molasses

Yes these are healthier choices when looking to add a touch of sweetness. However, they are still just sugars with minimal nutrients and need to be recognised as treats, not staples. Unless you have earned them with a high-intensity workout. Then you get to enjoy almost any sugar without any health consequences.

## What about fruit

However, fruit, in its original fresh form, should be enjoyed daily. There is no reason to restrict it any further than 2 pieces per day, if you exercise frequently, then you can often enjoy far more than that. Equally, you do not need to cut out carrots or sweet potato for fear of them being too sugary. The idea is ridiculous, based on a very simplistic view of how the body works.

## Summary

To summarise, you can enjoy sugars as a treat, if not abused then your body will tolerate them just fine. Sugars, just like other carbohydrates, fats and proteins, will be used to produce energy. Just remember that you use nutrients in the process of doing so, which is why they are treats.

However fruits are sources which come packaged with nutrients, therefore there's no nutrient deficit that results.

We must take our understanding of the language deeper than "Sugar = Bad" and understand that it is our body's control and tolerance of the sugar which is important. Many extremely healthy people in this world enjoy regular intake of fresh fruit salads with yoghurt, homemade treats sweetened with molasses, tea with honey and can even drizzle honey over their breakfast. Here's a snap of my favourite breakfast - my banana and tapioca flour crepes with fresh berries and raw organic honey.

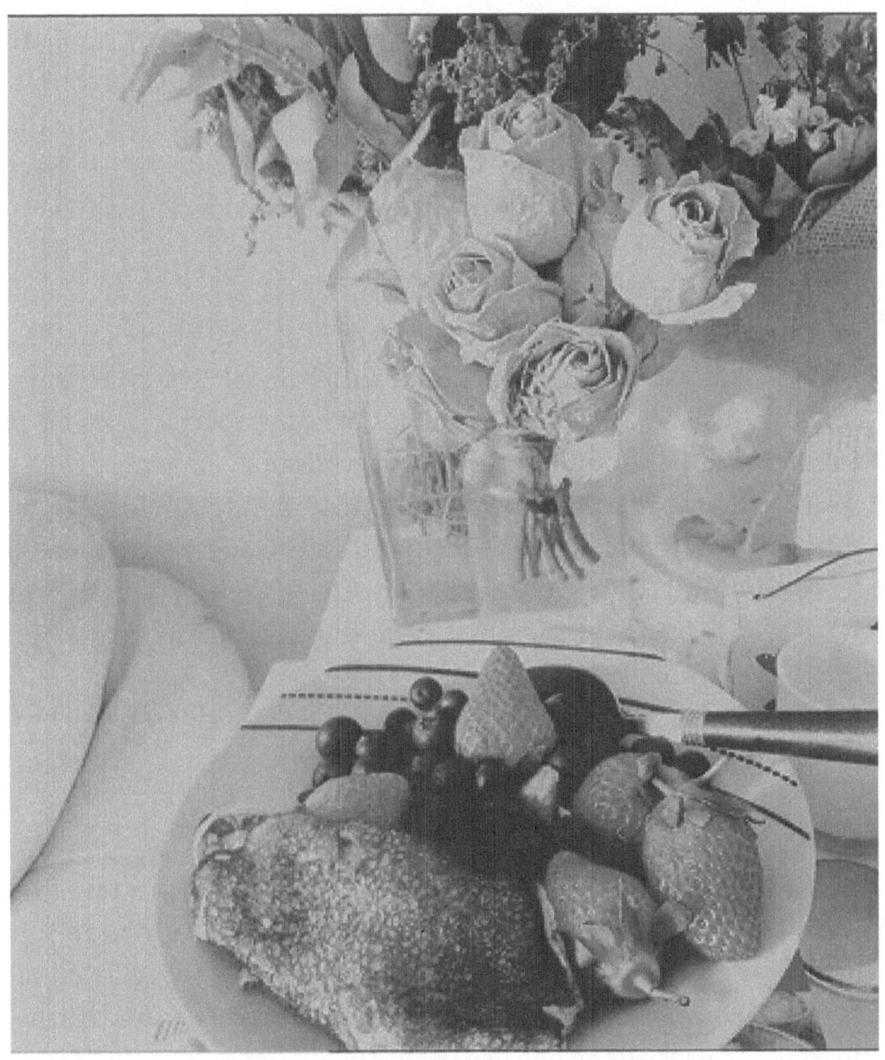

You too could be weird like me!

Adjust your diet to be more focused on healthy, unprocessed foods, and you'll be surprised how your palette changes. You'll find strawberries to be the sweetest thing you've ever tasted and will find commercial sweet treats to be overly sweet and quite frankly revolting.

I now mostly make my own treats, which is one of my favourite things to do. I sometimes flavour them with fresh fruit, sometimes with molasses or honey, sometimes with stevia. The fact is, now that my blood sugar is under control, I get to enjoy sugar as a treat, But it wasn't the sugar that was the problem to begin with, it was the way my body handled it.

Years ago I was diagnosed with polycystic ovarian syndrome or PCOS for short. This means that my body has an abnormal response to sugar (similar to diabetes) where it is difficult to tolerate sugar. In PCOS an excessive insulin response results from even small amounts of sugar. Typical complications are weight gain, acne, facial hair, infertility and awful PMS. I suffered from the acne and PMS while my blood sugar was poorly controlled. However, now I am entirely symptom-free, with very balanced hormones and a healthy tolerance of sugars.

Why is this? Did I need to go sugar-free to effect this change? No! Far from it in fact. What I needed was more efficient cells, more efficient hormonal (insulin) production.

By eating a whole food, low toxic chemical diet, I decrease the demand on my nutrient reserves. By reducing exposure to chemicals which attack and damage my cell walls, my blood sugar regulates naturally, my body is healthier, my energy production is more efficient, and my body uses all the glucose available to produce more and more energy.

My body now works just like it should. If I eat sugary foods such as banana or sweet potato, I get more energy, I'm stimulated to use it, and I burn it off. Sure I could abuse this system, go back to eating whole chocolate cakes and in time my body would be less efficient. But that's not the point here.

The point is, it is not going sugar-free that has improved the health of my patients or me.  It is eating a healthy diet, rich in nutrients, rich in fibre, protein, good quality fats.  It is eating natural sugars and knowing how to improve the body's tolerance and efficiency. It is using therapeutic foods which enhance the way our body absorbs and tolerates sugar, such as green tea, cacao and cinnamon.  It is recognising that sugar is a treat and enjoying it in moderation, not abusing it, but not cutting it out in a fad-like-fashion either.

## Review

So now that we've discussed this a little further, what's the verdict? Should you quit sugar for good?  Or should you work on removing processed, packaged, chemical-filled foods and replace them with natural, healthy, nutrient-rich foods, including naturally sugar-rich fruits, carrots and sweet potato?

# Week 3 Reflection

This week we have discussed many ways that our diet can be contributing to a toxic burden, resulting in poor health and decreased energy & happiness.

What was the biggest aha moment for you this week? Where will you begin?  If you are not yet eating a diet which is rich in fresh, healthy foods then "clean eating" may be a good goal to set as your primary focal point. Consider where your diet could do with the most assistance and begin making healthy swaps.

If your diet is already healthy, balanced and free of convenience foods and yet you're experiencing fatigue, digestive issues or simply interested in experimenting with further personalisation, then it may be time to experiment with reduced sugars or typically problematic foods to see if there are further improvements which could be made from additional modification.

Next week we move on to optimising sleep and correcting the diet for better energy. Your efforts this week will contribute to this and will determine how much of a benefit you experience from the additional practices added next week.

# VI

# Week 4: Getting better sleep

# The Benefits of Sleep

Last week we cleaned up our act, learned more about personalising our diet and by now you've hopefully got a good understanding of how to eat well to feel great. This week I'd like to build on this and work at optimising your well-being by improving one of our fundamental pillars of health - Sleep.

We've all felt the effects of a good night's sleep, and most of us have felt the awful effects of a restless or interrupted night.

Despite this, it seems to have become accepted that inadequate sleep is just something you have to live with. Very few people try to correct a poor sleep habit, or even know how to. Yet this is such a vital aspect of improving your health. Minimal improvements are felt until you fix this essential function.

So let's first look at why sleep is essential. To understand this, it's vital to discuss what happens during sleep.

Many people assume that sleep is like "Standby Mode" where we just shut down and stop using up energy so that there's energy to get up the next day. However, this is not true at all. In fact, sleep is one of our most active times, much more similar to a "System Recovery".

Sleep is where we begin our daily detox, begin repairing damaged tissues and also process the events of the day to decipher whether we are under threat and required to store energy (body fat) and conserve energy or are safe enough to grow, repair and expend energy as desired.

## What does this mean exactly?

It means that if you go to bed stressed, exhausted, over-stimulated, under-nourished or just too late in the day, your brain will determine you are under threat. The appropriate defences will be activated.

## Put simply:

- You will sleep less deeply, your body anxious that you may come under attack at any moment, poised and ready to fight.
- You will hold on to "fuel" and store energy so that we have these reserves to tap into as needed. You accumulate more body fat and crave more sugar.
- You will produce and use as little energy as possible throughout the day so that reserves stay full. Available energy feels low, all systems run slower, we move less, brain function slows metabolism slows, and the digestive system may shut down (think constipation). You feel tired, lethargic, unmotivated, sleepy, less hungry yet craving sugar and of course, are constipated.
- Stress hormones will be on the starting block, ready to activate at a moments notice. This means you are more jumpy, less grounded, less rational and more likely to "over-react" or make poor decisions.
- You will fear activities which further reduce energy such as exercise, socialising, learning or creating change.

## The alternative:

Inversely, when you go to bed calm, content, well fed (think nutrients not calories here) and with adequate time for quality sleep, your brain will determine that you are safe. This means it is now safe to commence growth, repair, appropriate metabolism and to use as much energy as is desired to do so.

## What this means:

- You will sleep deeply and calmly, your brain will begin scanning your body for damaged tissues which require repair and program your body to be more efficient the following day at any tasks which have been practiced today.
- Your body will begin rebuilding and repairing muscles, organs, skin and eyes as required.
- You will expend as much energy as necessary to complete all essential healing/detox/recovery.
- You will process the events of your day and determine a rational response. The memories and thoughts will now be processed and stored as part of learning.

## How you'll feel:

- You will wake feeling refreshed, energised, calm and ready for your day.
- You will be capable of learning and processing new information without feeling overwhelmed.
- You will be capable of responding rationally and calmly to any events or challenges.
- You will have unrestricted access to your energy reserves and will not fear duties which use this energy such as exercise, socialising,

adapting or learning new behaviours.

- Your metabolism, immune system and digestive system will have all the energy it needs to perform at it's best.

So now you can see why a good night's sleep is so important. Hopefully, this has inspired you to prioritise this area. Now let's discuss my top 5 techniques for improving sleep plus what I do to assist the "problem" or chronic cases and for children with special needs where standard methods fail.

## Tip 1: Reduce stimulants and support your sleep & energy naturally

This is an essential and necessary first step. Start by limiting yourself to no sugar, caffeine or chocolate after 2pm - yes this includes dark chocolate (the most stimulating). To support your energy throughout the day, B Vitamins work best. They assist your body in producing more energy while also regulating sleep cycles.

I also recommend taking a natural medicine for sleep support. Magnesium works really well here. However, there are also excellent herbal formulas containing Zyziphus and Lavender extract that help you to wind down from the stress of the day with the added benefit of boosting your production of Melatonin. This offers improved sleep with no drowsiness the next day, in fact, I often find myself more alert and motivated the following day which reduces the need for the coffee which leads to better sleep.. and so the cycle continues.

## Tip 2: Do the right type of exercise (at the right time)

Exercise is a great way to improve your sleep, but it must be the right type of activity at the right time of day. Yoga, Pilates and Swimming are the best forms of exercise for the evening as they are calming and initiate the parasympathetic nervous system or the "rest and digest" response.

Aerobic exercise, HIIT, heavy weight training, cross fit and dance classes are best served earlier in the day. These types of exercise help to initiate an energising release of "happy chemicals" which make you feel inspired, excited and generally happy to be alive. This works well before work or at lunchtime but if practised in the evening may result in you being overstimulated and lying awake buzzing with ideas. We've all been there.

## Tip 3: Reduce stress-inducing activities at night

This means not checking your finances/writing your to-do list/watching the news/checking up on your ex's social media feed/watching a scary movie/discussing things which may cause arguments with your partner or housemate/paying bills in the evening before bed. If any of the above must be done, do them well before bedtime and then move on to Tip 4.

## Tip 4: Introduce a calming, stress busting, soothing routine that prepares you for sleep

This could be a hot shower with lavender oil, a meditation session or a light yin yoga session. I often get my patients to use a meditation app such as Calm, Yoga Studio or HeadSpace to help completely relax before sleep. It's highly effective, even for the most tightly wound.

## Tip 5: Plan for sleep

It might sound funny but an essential factor to consider when you are trying to improve sleep is actually to make sleep a high priority. Let sleep become what your evening is all about! Sleep is hardly ever going to improve when it is seen as an inconvenience that must be put off until the last moment as you're suffering from evening FOMO (fear of missing out). Let your evening be a gradual warm up towards a deep and relaxing sleep. Sleep is something to be celebrated, nurtured and prioritised. Let your rest be the reward for a busy day, not the payment.

# Caffeine & Sugar on Sleep

## Caffeine

Caffeine initiates a stress response in most people which results in an energy surge conserved for running away from danger. This process, known as the fight or flight stage, also inhibits digestion. Only when the "rest and digest" phase kicks in are you able to absorb vital nutrients from your food.

Many people have a restless, disturbed or poor quality sleep when under the influence of caffeine from coffee or energy drinks. Inversely, green tea has a calming effect, due to containing Theanine, an incredible nutrient which is calming and initiates the parasympathetic nervous system known as the "rest and digest" response. Therefore, even though some green teas such as matcha contain caffeine, the balance of caffeine vs theanine allows you to enjoy a hot cuppa without any adverse effects.

Green tea as a bitter food also increases vital digestive enzymes, kick starts liver detox pathways, improves sugar metabolism and can regulate appetite. But we'll come to that in later weeks as we discuss these details in single focus.

Many people are sensitive to caffeine. For them, even one morning-coffee is enough to disturb sleep later that night. Coffee consumption also depletes magnesium; our primary relaxation mineral which also regulates the digestive system and controls blood sugar.

If you would like to improve sleep, I would highly recommend reducing your caffeine consumption to as little as possible. If you are able to cut the coffee altogether and switch to green tea, then I'd highly recommend this. You may feel worse initially, for 3 days or so but after that, you'll start to feel better and better. Your sleep will improve, your energy will be your own (rather than borrowed energy that must be repaid later), and your appetite will be more controlled.

If you are unable or unwilling to cut your coffee altogether, I'd recommend having just the 1 coffee at 9am. At this stage your breakfast should be mostly digested, your stress hormones balanced and your body reasonably hydrated. This makes the effects of the coffee less detrimental. Please refrain from having more than 1 cup per day and never have coffee past 12pm (unless of course, you are using it to stay awake all night you party animal).

## Sugar

It's not uncommon to suffer sugar cravings at night after dinner. In fact, the more stressed you are, the stronger the sugar cravings typically are.

It's important to remember that sugar's role is to provide energy. At night, we want to be calming ourselves in preparation for sleep. Having a sugar hit before bed may inhibit a restful sleep as the dopamine surge may increase excitement. A much better choice is to stick with a piece of fresh fruit, some veggie sticks with hummus or almond butter, or even just a camomile tea.

Some people do find that a cup of warm milky tea with honey provides a better quality sleep. This is primarily due to the memory of the soothing, comforting and nurturing experience of breast milk, a memory which stays with us subconsciously throughout our lives. However getting the recipe right here is essential. It's vital to ensure that you don't over-excite yourself, or crowd out the melatonin. See the recipes section for a tea that will help you sleep, while also supporting an over-night detox.

# Protein for Sleep

dequate protein supply throughout the day is essential for good sleep. If you are experiencing insomnia for no good reason, it is possible that you are not consuming adequate protein each day.

I've found that many of my problem sleepers respond really well to taking larger amounts of protein at dinner time. This works particularly well when combined with anti-inflammatory fats which reduce stress.

The protein based meals which appear to have the most significant effect are:

- A palm-sized serve of Salmon with green veggies and 2 small potatoes dressed in olive oil.
- A protein smoothie (I usually recommend a rice or hemp-based protein powder) with half a banana and flaxseed oil.
- Fermented grain bread topped with avocado, olives and pumpkin seeds.
- Dahl and brown rice

Protein supplies many essential amino acids which assist with promoting a deep, restorative sleep. We do the bulk of our repair work, detox and growing at night. This is where protein really shines. An adequate supply of good quality protein means plenty of essential amino acids to support this repair work, protect the liver during detox and to provide the building blocks for tissue growth.

It is easy to get enough protein each day. A healthy, balanced diet generally supplies adequate amounts for the average person.

Some people respond well to taking a serve of protein right before bed.  For this, I usually recommend an alkalising, vegan protein powder mixed with coconut water (further alkalising), a serve of meat, fish or eggs. I'd recommend experimenting with a few sources until you find the one which works best for you.

# Routine & Regular Bed Times

It may sound silly, but creating a regular bedtime and routine are two of the most essential and useful practices for improving your sleep. We respond very well to routine and having a night time routine that prepares us for rest can be more effective than any sleeping pill.

There are a couple of things that I usually recommend to my patients. When you hear them, you'll realise how commonsense and straightforward they are, yet few of us naturally do them. Our night time routine is entirely upside down.

### The evening routine

Firstly I want you to think about what the first thing you do in the morning to wake yourself up is. You wash your face and brush your teeth, right? How much more awake do you feel with your clean face and minty fresh breath? It feels good, doesn't it?

Now I want you to think about the last thing you do at night, right before you climb into bed and try to settle in for a good night's sleep. You probably wash your face and brush your teeth, don't you? We all do! This is one of the first things that needs to change.

Now I should preface this by saying that if you're tired, relaxed and ready for bed with no concerns about how much sleep you're able to get. You'll probably fall asleep regardless. But how hard do you think it's going to be to fall asleep with the fresh taste of peppermint in your mouth, particularly when you're already feeling restless, stressed or suffering sleep issues.

This week I'd like you to try something for me. After dinner, I'd like you to head to the bathroom, wash your face, brush your teeth, shower, take care of your entire nighttime hygiene routine. Then change into some cozy pyjamas and carry on with your evening.

The beautiful thing about moving your evening hygiene routine to an earlier time is that you not only prepare your body and mind for an earlier sleep, you actually start to relax much more too. Often my patients report that, where previously they had sat watching TV until late hours of the evening, they now found themselves voluntarily going to bed earlier to read as they have started to crave the relaxation time. This is a really significant shift and one which creates a substantial change in your body clock.

## Regular bedtimes

The second important practice for improving your night's sleep is to have regular bedtimes. When you take yourself off to bed at a similar time each night, you'll find it's easier to fall asleep naturally, your body clock expects it. Also, you'll find it easier to wake without an alarm and will feel more rested on waking as you'll have trained your biological clock to respond this way naturally.

Often when I discuss this idea, many of my patients ask "what about weekends". Here I think it's important first to determine what is most important. If you enjoy staying out late, enjoy any activities or work a job which requires you to stay up late on weekends then yes we need to work around this. However, if you're simply staying up later on weekends to watch tv, then you're probably doing so out of a childlike "because I can" attitude.

This really kicked in for me when I left my job to work for myself. My working hours had meant an enforced wake up time of 6am, 5 days per week for the past 5 years. Now working for myself and only practising 2 days per week, I was back in complete control of my bedtime. In fact, I could afford to stay up past midnight any day of the week. Even if I stayed up very late the night before work, it wouldn't really matter too much as I had only 1 day at work before at least 1 more day off to sleep in, nap or rest. I revelled in the rebellion, and it felt fabulous.

However, it wasn't long before I started feeling tired again most days. I stopped enjoying exercise and found it difficult to get myself to the gym, even though I now had so much free time. I also started craving sugary foods and caffeine again. All of this was due to my inconsistent bedtimes. It was time to make a change. I re-established a healthy evening routine, designed to promote healthy and restorative sleep, and was feeling rested, refreshed and energetic again in no time.

## But what about the weekends?

The truth is, after some evaluating, I realised that on weekends, what I enjoyed most was waking up feeling refreshed, having a small sleep in (rarely past 8am I should mention) and then getting up and getting out to enjoy the day. Sure it's nice to stay up late occasionally if I need to, but mostly I get to bed at the same time on weekends as through the week. The daytime is most important to me, and it is not worth throwing out my whole week's sleep, just to stay up an extra few hours.

Mind you 21 year old Jen wouldn't have agreed, she stayed up at all costs. Even if it meant no sleep at all. At 21 I had severe FOMO and never wanted to go to bed, even though there was rarely anything really worth staying up for. Ultimately this led to overuse of stimulants and worsened the chronic fatigue, leading to depression, a lack of emotional resilience and feeling generally vulnerable and weak. This is part of the reason that she did not leave the unsafe environment she was living in, the alternative just seemed too stressful and she pure and simple did not have the energy or strength to make a move – until there was no choice. But we'll come back to that.

# Bedtime Meditation & Relaxation

Now that we've discussed the ideal evening routine. Let's talk through bedtime itself.

You've now taken all the right steps, you've eaten well but not too much. Have had a serve of protein, are well hydrated, have taken time to relax, had your shower and brushed your teeth hours ago. You're ready for bed.

So now it's time to get into bed, what now? What if you still can't get to sleep? There are a few fall-back plans and sleep enhancers which can greatly assist.

Follow my 3 step plan below for the ultimate in indulgent bedtimes. If you're still awake at the end of step 3, just appreciate the luxury of having more time to enjoy it:

## Step 1: Aromatherapy

Take some lavender oil or jasmine and sprinkle a few drops on your quilt and pillow. Don't over-fragrance here, it's important to be smart. If you go crazy with the scent, it will irritate your airways and possibly have the opposite effect. Just a few drops are enough.

Both lavender and jasmine oils are aromatherapy oils which help to calm and soothe, promoting muscle relaxation and calm.

## Step 2: Releasing the day

Now it's time to climb into that heavenly scented bed and take some time to release the day. Give yourself permission to be fully absorbed in the feeling of being held by your bed. Appreciate the softness of your pillow, enjoy the feeling of being supported by your mattress.

Allow yourself now to let go. Let go of any disappointments, frustrations or tensions. If thoughts of other people creep in here, release them also. Tell yourself "not now, this is MY time!". Take this time entirely for yourself. If you've ever attended a yoga class you'll know this feeling, this is your Shavasana. As one of my favourite yogis' once instructed - Don't miss this!

Any time your mind wanders, remind yourself "don't miss this". It's really quite a delicious feeling to be wrapped in a bed, with nowhere to be than right here. We just over-complicate things. Allow yourself to feel it for all it's worth right now.

## Step 3: Meditation

You can do this using an app such as Headspace or Calm, you could even use a Calm sleep story. Alternatively, you can use the tried and tested body scan.

## Body Scan:

Start at the feet, focusing on the toes and the muscles at the top of the feet. Focus on relaxing them now, take some deep breaths as you do breathing in and out through the nose. Move through the body, from the tip of the toes to the head, relaxing every muscle consciously as you reach it. Enjoy the sensation of relaxing and being absorbed by your bed.

# Week 4 Reflection

This week we focused our attention on the benefits of sleep. How do you feel about these changes?

I hope that you've begun to experience some benefits from the changes we've implemented and are starting to see your energy recover. Next week we will expand on this further by modifying our diet and lifestyle for better stress resilience, which should also help to promote better sleep.

However, before we move on, it's important to recognise that all attempts to correct your stress are futile if we are not getting good quality sleep, as exhaustion makes stress more stressful.

So, before we close this week, let's set some SMART goals for continuing to work on our sleep. What next steps can you commit to?

Examples include:

- Could you reduce your caffeine or sugar intake to prevent over-stimulation?
- Could you improve on your protein intake, or increase your serve at night time (without overeating)?
- Could you improve on your evening routine to set yourself up for quality sleep
- Could you introduce some bedtime meditation practices to calm

your nervous system?

Whatever goals you choose, remember to keep them small, measurable, agreed upon, realistic and time measured. Setting SMART goals prevents overwhelm and allows you to build each week without undoing any of your hard work.

# VII

# Week 5: Reducing anxiety & stress

# Are You Stressed?

Over the last few weeks, we have incorporated many dietary and lifestyle changes to improve our health and happiness. Last week we focused on sleep and discussed some routines, regimens, removals and reductions we could make to enhance the quality of our sleep. Hopefully, this is already helping you to feel a little less stressed and a little more healthy and happy.

Now it's time to focus on an area which often undoes all of our good work. For some this week may be the most significant. Do you feel that all your efforts so far are just to counterbalance the major stressors in your life? If so this week is for you my friend. Let's talk Stress!

## Stress the great Undo-er

Stress is known universally amongst healthcare practitioners as "The Great Undo-er". Stress at its peak wipes away all of your hard work each day, your efforts are merely damage control, beneficial in the short term, but like climbing a stair-master, you're going nowhere!

There is no end of research displaying the positive effects of a healthy diet, exercise and meditation on stress. We know that when we eat better, exercise, sleep well and take time to meditate, we feel better, and life feels less stressful.

Today we're going to cover the foundations of what is actually happening during the stress response, what it is triggered by and how we can turn it all around. I'm going to give you a couple of tools to implement which will help you manage your stress more effectively and discuss specific pathways you can take to minimise stress and begin healing quickly.

## The stress response - Fight or flight

The stress response is perfectly designed to help you to run away from, or fight danger. It is known as the "fight or flight" response. In its correct form, when used for this purpose, to run away from danger, it is highly beneficial.

However, when sitting at your work desk, shovelling in a quick salad in an attempt to nourish your body during a busy and stressful workday, the restriction of blood flow, enzymes and signalling to your digestive system leads to poor digestion and inability to absorb nutrients. Over time this leads to nutritional deficiencies and a digestive system which is dysfunctional.

The immune system, which becomes hypersensitive during the stress response is a protective measure to improve your healing capacity. However, when stress is prolonged, this can leave you more prone to food sensitivities and other allergic reactions.

While the fight or flight response was designed to help us escape or fight, the rest and digest response is the opposite. Consider yourself running away from a predator, while fight or flight assists you to run away, there must be a resting phase that kicks in once you have reached safety. While both play vital roles in our survival, it is this resting phase which many of us are lacking and are suffering many health issues as a consequence.

## The rest and digest phase

The parasympathetic nervous system, known as the "rest and digest" response, kicks in following a stressful event to allow us to relax and recover our strength. We now feel calm and enjoy a heightened endorphin (happy chemical) rush to assist us in recognising how beautiful it is to be alive and to ensure we think that all the hard work (running) was worth it. Healing, growing, adapting and learning is now safe to begin.

## Short term vs Chronic Stress

In the short term, stress, as seen with exercise or watching a scary movie, can be perfectly harmless. We flick from fight or flight to rest and digest with ease and recover well. We feel stimulated by the stress as it forced us to push through barriers we were not sure we could break, and we feel a sense of achievement for having survived unscathed.

However long-term, severe or chronic stress can be highly detrimental. You lose your "off switch" as your rest and digest phase is rarely stimulated. You run on stress hormones, flicking from exhausted to overstimulated and anxious, rushing through your life running on fumes and progressively losing your resilience. All the while you are reducing your ability to heal, recover or grow.

If you have experienced severe stress or trauma, particularly in your developmental years, then there are physical changes and adaptations in your body's response to stress. For some this can lead to severe anger or chronic anxiety, for others this can lead to chronic fatigue and feeling exhausted from any stressful event, no matter how small. This leads to multiple complications which we will discuss further shortly. First, let's discuss the drivers of stress.

## Focus Point 1: Identifying stressors in your life

There are many causes of stress, just being too busy is a common one. However, we expect to push through again and again with little rest or recovery time. We assume that a sleep-in, a sick day, a lazy weekend or a week or two on a beachy holiday will put us right again. However, this only deals with the top layer - low energy. Many of the underlying layers are left untouched.

Identifying causes or triggers of stress can allow us to set a plan for re-structuring, re-prioritising and re-organising our responsibilities. This leads to more energy for healing, more motivation for new and exciting introductions to our life, and a happier, well-balanced self that feels ready for any challenge we may have to face.

## Step 1: Identify any significant causes of stress

- Personal and family issues
- Work-related pressures
- Financial pressures
- Divorce, separation or relationship breakdown
- Unstable foundations: moving home / work / someone you love moving away
- Death of a loved one
- Injury and illness

These issues are all significant causes of stress, going through any of the above is a substantial drain on your energy and emotional stability. Experiencing one or more will leave you depleted of valuable nutrients, with a reduced ability to heal and more susceptible to adverse stress reactions while your body recovers.

## Step 2: Identify other triggers of stress

Many of the following have a significant impact, despite being less commonly known. Such as:

- Hormonal imbalances
- Nutritional deficiencies
- Food Intolerances
- Dehydration
- Inflammation
- High caffeine or excessive sugar intake
- Candida overgrowth
- Poor sleep quality
- Medications such as antibiotics, antihistamines, the contraceptive pill
- Lack of exercise
- Lack of time outdoors: low vitamin D levels, low ocular photo-stimulation (natural light in the eyes), low oxygen intake

These causes are less recognised and may often go unnoticed. By taking a moment to identify any significant stressors, you understand yourself a little better. You can understand the emotional and physical load which you have been under, and understand why your health may not be at it's best. By understanding other mild stressors which may be exacerbating the problem and inhibiting your recovery, we can determine the necessary steps to take to restore your body to full health.

## Are you feeling stressed?

Addressing, and taking measures to counteract stress must be a vital component of any healthy living program. Stress increases our demand for crucial nutrients, yet decreases the ability to absorb them. Stress also leads to lowered immunity, which may detract you from your health goals for a week or more.  More importantly, chronic and/or severe stress increases your risk of almost every major disease, and therefore must be addressed to live a healthy, happy life.

Often our perception of how stressed we are is very relative. Therefore if we feel less stressed than we did 1 year ago, we may think that our life is well balanced. However this may not be the case, an effective measure for identifying stress is to look for the physical signs.

If you are experiencing sugar cravings, anxiety, insomnia, reduced energy, shaky hands, inability to concentrate, stubborn weight gain around your middle, persistent bloating despite removing your problem foods, desire to retreat from your responsibilities or feel that you just can't switch off effectively, taking measures to reduce stress will be highly beneficial for you.

## What can we do about it?

First, the most beneficial way to begin breaking this cycle is to identify the stressors in your life. We'll address this shortly in the health and happiness questionnaire. This will allow you to take an objective look at what can be done to create the necessary change. This is the first step in reclaiming your body and mind.

We can then begin working on the required changes. These may be changes which you can comfortably make on your own, or you may need assistance from someone who can walk you through a step by step action plan. Remember to ask for help when needed.

There may be stressors that do not have any immediate solution. In this instance, the key is to identify them and to identify factors which we can use to reduce the negative consequence of stress.

For example;

If you feel stressed because your work is going through a major restructure, and you are not sure that your job is stable, then there is little we can do to resolve this. However, we must recognise that this is having an adverse effect on your health, even in the short term, and therefore must do something to counteract this.

In this instance, you may be required to work longer hours and/or through your lunch break, may find the work environment more draining and intense during those hours. This is going to increase your production of cortisol and adrenaline. This will deplete your magnesium and B vitamins, amongst other things.

Being stressed over lunchtime and eating at your desk, may lead to poor digestion, leading to nutrient deficiencies, leading to further stress and fatigue.

## Solution 1:

Plan ahead for healthy, easily digestible meals that can be eaten in 10 minutes or less. Good examples are soups, salads and smoothies. Be sure to add plenty of omega 3 fats, our calming, anti-inflammatory fats. The alkalising foods will also help to calm the consequence of stress.

## Solution 2:

If possible, take 10 minutes to meditate before eating lunch. Using an app such as Calm or Headspace, you can sit quietly with your headphones in and meditate literally anywhere. If you can't get any access to a quiet space then go to the bathroom and do this while sitting on the toilet. However, it is much more effective if you can take a moment to sit outside.

Solution 3:

Take a calming, restorative supplement and incorporate herbal teas. If you're particularly stressed and anxious, then drinking chamomile tea throughout the day can be particularly beneficial.  Green tea offers the stimulation of a mild caffeine boost, coupled with the calming effect of the Epigallocatechin Gallate (**EGCG**) which soothes and eases the stress response.  Green tea also offers a detox boost, improves production of digestive enzymes and is full of antioxidants for beautiful clear skin.

By putting in place these solutions, we improve our body's capability of healing from the negative consequences of stress. By taking time to prepare, we prevent the stressful, busy time from having further negative implications by driving unhealthy choices. With meditation, we build better resilience, a calmer, more objective, peaceful mind and greater coping skills overall. in short, while we have not rid ourselves of the stress, we have improved our emotional and physical tolerance so it now has less of an impact on our well-being.

The Pure Health & Happiness protocol to reduce (and recover from) stress:
- Heal your body with a nourishing diet which will replenish lost nutrients.  The Pure Health & Happiness diet is ideal for stress recovery.
- Eat slowly and more mindfully, take time to enjoy your meal. Appreciate the flavours and textures, let food be your medicine. I call this meditative eating, we'll discuss this shortly.
- Prioritise sleep and create a low-stress sleep environment. Hopefully you've started feeling the benefits of this since last week.
- Meditate. A practice of 10 minutes of daily meditation or mindful-

ness training is demonstrated to enhance recovery from emotional and physical stress. Meditation assists you to manage stress more appropriately, to make essential decisions more easily and to restore deficient energy levels. We'll discuss this further shortly

· Take time out for fun: Something we often let go during busy and stressful times. Make (alcohol free) fun a priority at least 1 day per week. Ideas: trampolining, dance class, art class, head to the beach, play with your pet/children etc.

· Reduce caffeine. Focus on the natural methods for boosting energy which encourage, rather than inhibit, the recovery from stress. We'll discuss energy further next week.

· Finally, drink more tea! [7]

Note: If your stress is ongoing or severe, or you're finding it a challenge to recover. Consider consulting a Nutritionist to determine the appropriate supplements you should be taking. Formulas containing healing medicines such as ginseng, B Complex Vitamins and Magnesium are incredibly powerful during times of stress. However a Nutrition professional can guide you towards the ideal support for you. Remember there's always my Comprehensive Health Screening (see final page) if you'd like a whole-health assessment and personalised prescription.[8]

---

[7] Green tea regulates the sleep-wake cycle, improves liver detox and contains Theanine, a calming amino acid which reduces stress. Camomile tea is wonderfully calming and can assist with promoting a good nights sleep. If you feel stressed at work, try a green and jasmine tea which will provide you with clarity, focus, energy and a sense of calm all at once (jasmine is a calming, aromatherapy herb). Lavender tea is another beautiful option - very calming and can actually assist with rebalancing the good and bad bacteria in your digestive system.

[8] I typically assess each patient to determine the most appropriate supplement for them, based on how their body is responding to the stress. This support can really assist in taking the edge off and helping you to enjoy life (and all of its challenges) once again.

# Health & Happiness Questionnaire

Let's now take a moment to complete the health and happiness questionnaire. This will assist in drawing attention to the key areas which need attention, and to identify how stress is currently impacting our health, happiness and general well-being. The aim is to score 10 points or more. However the most important step right now is to establish a baseline which you can continue to work on and review throughout this program.

*For every question you answer yes give yourself 1 point:*

1. Do you consider yourself to be happy?
2. Do you wake with energy?
3. Do you feel motivated to exercise?
4. Do you feel supported by your friendships?
5. Do you feel loved by your family?
6. Do you feel valued in your job?
7. Do you sleep easily and wake refreshed?
8. Do you have a hobby?
9. Do you regularly participate in fun activities that do not involve alcohol or illicit drugs?
10. Do you know your value within your family/community/work?
11. Re: above, do you feel that others value your contribution?
12. Do you have a place you can feel calm and safe? Do you have a sanctuary of peace?
13. Do you have a space you can go when you need to be creative?

14. Do you know what energises and motivates you?


*Now, for every question you answer yes to the following, deduct 2 points:*

1. Do you feel useless or hopeless or are others telling you this?
2. Do you experience times where you feel overstimulated and desire to be able to retreat to a dark, quiet space?
3. Do you feel anxious?
4. Do you suffer from insomnia?
5. Do you rely on caffeine for motivation?
6. Do you rely on alcohol to calm you down?
7. Do you suffer from night time sweet cravings?
8. Do you experience nightmares?
9. Do you suffer from depression?
10. Do you avoid social interaction?
11. Do you experience anxiety or phobia when stepping out of your comfort zone?

# What Are Your Priorities?

By answering the questions in the health and happiness questionnaire, you now have an idea of the key areas which need focus. So now let me ask you, how healthy and happy are you?

I've provided a scoring system to tell you what I would aim for with you to be but this is your journey and your goal. Are you happy with your current choices? Do you want to change? Do you want to experience a higher level of health?

My suggestion would be to highlight those key areas that have been identified in this questionnaire to be letting you down. Begin now organising them by order of priority. Be smart about this and choose wisely.

For best results, have your completed questionnaire reviewed by your Nutritionist or Naturopath. A health professional can help you to organise the changes by order of priority, and create a step-by-step action plan which will help you to improve your mental and general health.

For example:

Let's say you are currently crawling out of bed exhausted, drinking 2-3 coffees or energy drinks throughout the day, battling IBS, suffering anxiety and insomnia and then repeating this cycle daily. Let's say your goal is to increase your exercise, cut back on sugar and lose weight. How successful do you think you will be in making the change without first addressing the energy imbalance?

To me when I see this cycle (an all too common occurrence in my practice), I know that the excess caffeine is driving your anxiety and keeping you awake at night, reducing the quality of your sleep in general, which of course is driving your fatigue on rising.

The resultant surge in stress hormones is also over-stimulating your digestive system (think nervous poos) and energy pathways (think energy high followed by a crash), so you are losing nutrients quicker than you are able to replace them.

The fatigue is driving more coffee and sugar cravings, and you feel out of control of your emotions, energy and appetite. You want to change, but your body is in panic and is overriding your decisions in an attempt to survive.

So you see, aiming for more exercise and less sugar as your first step is not an achievable goal. You need to cut the coffee first but you're exhausted, how will you do it?

As a Nutritionist, I'd give you a multivitamin with a good dose of B Vitamins which help to naturally boost energy production. Unlike coffee which simply increases your use of energy (think of pedal to the metal), B Vitamins help to refuel the tank with energy efficient fuel. They also help with liver detoxification, are necessary for the production of red blood cells (which deliver oxygen to your brain and muscles) and help to regulate your sleep-wake cycles.

I'd also prescribe an Alpha-Lipoic-Acid formula which would help to improve your sugar metabolism while also boosting energy, and would advise you of energy boosting foods to include at breakfast and lunch.

Finally, I would put in place a plan for caffeine reduction and would help to work towards resuming exercise in time with the naturally increased energy.  Now you are sleeping better, rising with energy and no longer craving sugar or starchy carbohydrates. You are more likely to respond well to exercise, will recover more easily and will look forward to your sessions making it easier to form a healthy habit.

# Neurotransmitters

The reason the Pure Health and Happiness program makes you feel happier is due to the impact on your neurotransmitters.

## What are Neurotransmitters?

Neurotransmitters are sometimes nicknamed "chemicals" or "happy hormones". Neither are really correct. In fact, they are chemical messengers which deliver important information and play a major role in our everyday life and our body's major functions. Your neurotransmitter balance determines your sleep, appetite, metabolism as well as your mood, stress tolerance and pain perception.

There are some neurotransmitters which you may be familiar with, others may be very new to you. In this chapter, I'm going to cover the basics of the ones which have the strongest impact on your health and happiness.

## Serotonin

Serotonin is a neurotransmitter which instils a sense of peace, happiness and calm. In the gastrointestinal tract (where 90% of our serotonin is found), serotonin regulates our bowel movements.

When our serotonin is in balance, we have good stress tolerance, a good outlook on life, enjoy healthy and easy bowel movements and generally experience less unhealthy cravings.

When serotonin is low, we may experience anxiety, poor sleep, constipation, low energy, low mood and cravings for sugar or starchy carbohydrates.

Serotonin is also used to make melatonin, the hormone which puts us into a deep, restorative sleep. This is why, when our serotonin is low, we may also experience insomnia, fatigue and/or restless sleep. Nightmares are also quite common.

Our body manufactures serotonin from tryptophan, an amino acid which we get from foods high in protein. Foods rich in tryptophan include eggs, fish, soybeans, sunflower and sesame seeds.

## Dopamine

The neurotransmitter dopamine plays a major role in our reward-motivated behaviours such as eating, competing and sex. It boosts our focus, motivation and concentration.

Dopamine also plays a major role in our insulin response (the hormone that controls blood sugar), controls our cardiovascular system, our control of our salts and the control of our muscles.

One of the reasons we enjoy eating, particularly sugary or chocolate based foods, is that it increases dopamine release. It is, in fact, often the dopamine that we are addicted to rather than the food itself. This is also the key behind compulsive, binge and emotional eating - the ongoing search for dopamine.

When in balance, dopamine makes us feel wonderful. We are happy, motivated and focused. We feel a sense of achievement and satisfaction. We are able to work towards goals. When out of balance however, we feel flat, apathetic and out of control. We suffer sleep issues and lose concentration very easily. In short, we lose our zest for life.

Have you noticed how much more motivated you are after a cup of coffee? That's also down to the resultant dopamine response. This is fine if occasional, or if we are happy and healthy. However, relying on this false stimulation can lead to devastating effects. Have you noticed how the coffee becomes less effective and how it takes more and more cups to get you going? This is when you're starting to hit trouble.

If abused, with high caffeine intake or illegal dopamine-inducing substances (or chronic stress), your dopamine receptors will become less responsive. Your dopamine release may reduce, and you'll feel fatigued and unmotivated as a result.

In time, all types of reward-motivated behaviour no longer stimulate you. You'll be apathetic about sex, uninterested in competing in any way, may lose interest in your job and one of two things may happen with your diet.

Some people at this stage lose all interest in eating, there is no pleasure felt from anything. Others eat more, searching for the dopamine release they are sure will come. Some can be seen eating a whole chocolate cake and feeling no pleasure, continuing until they feel positively sick... believe me this is not a fun place to be.

Dopamine is synthesised from the amino acid Tyrosine which we get from protein, therefore our dietary balance plays a big role here. Healthy ways to stimulate dopamine release include healthy balanced meals rich in protein, leafy greens, nuts, seeds and avocados.

Occasional coffee consumption and consuming superfoods such as matcha or raw cacao are also ways to get a healthy dopamine boost. As a Nutritionist, I'm lucky enough to be able to prescribe to my patients nutrients such as N-Acetyl-Cysteine which improve and promote healthy dopamine release in a matter of days.

And let's not forget of course exercise, which, when coupled with a healthy, protein-rich diet, stimulates the release of dopamine. By providing tyrosine-rich foods to your body, you increase your production, by exercising you stimulate the release, a winning combination wouldn't you say? Translation: A healthy balanced diet plus exercise = leaving the gym high on dopamine, feeling like a champ. Unhealthy diet plus exercise = leaving feeling exhausted and often wondering why you bother.

## GABA

Now here's one you may not have heard of before. GABA is an unsung hero worthy of serious worship. In fact, we owe many of our greatest accomplishments to this wonderful neurotransmitter.

GABA is short for Gamma-Aminobutyric-Acid. Let's just stick with the acronym, shall we?

GABA is our anti-anxiety neurotransmitter. It reduces sensitivity to pain, regulates stress, improves sleep quality and controls muscle tone. GABA release is the reason you feel calm after a good meditation session, it is the hero that stops your panic attack escalating during stressful events and is the reason you are still capable of performing under stress.

GABA is made from glutamate (a neurotransmitter which excites, rather than calms you) using specific enzymes and cofactors such as vitamin B6.

When running low in GABA, we may suffer insomnia, anxiety, social phobia and/or depression.

In my clinic, I often use a compounded form of GABA for my patients to assist with chronic stress, pain, insomnia or anxiety. I also increase fermented foods such as sauerkraut and kimchi which are food sources of GABA.

## Histamine

Histamine is best known for its immunomodulatory role in the allergy response. High histamine response in response to an immune challenge or allergy is typically experienced as hives, itchy rash, hayfever symptoms or, in extreme cases, anaphylaxis.

It has become very common for people to take a regular dose of anti-histamines, which in some cases is absolutely necessary in order to maintain health. However, anti-histamines affect the brain too, where it acts as a neurotransmitter.

The neurotransmitter histamine prevents sleep and is excitatory. Increased histamine production may, therefore, lead to anxiety and insomnia. Antihistamines bind to the histamine receptors, preventing histamine from attaching. However, this does not prevent the body from producing histamine, and the blood can become flooded. Over time, the body becomes less responsive to anti-histamines and, due to the large amount in circulation, the effects of histamine are often now much pronounced.

In short, histamine makes you itchy, irritable, anxious and prevents sleep. Antihistamines such as Benadryl knock you out by blocking the receptors. However, they do not reduce histamine production. Newer, non-drowsy antihistamines, do not block the receptors in the central nervous system and therefore only act on the receptors in the gut and those involved in the immune response.

There are many anti-histamine foods and nutrients which are a safe and effective way to reduce hives, hayfever and allergy symptoms without the resultant effects in the brain. Nutrients such as vitamin C, found in citrus fruits such as lemons, grapefruit and oranges have an anti-histamine effect. Quercetin is another antihistamine nutrient which is found in red kidney beans, radish, coriander, onions and dill.

There are many more neurotransmitters which control the complicated and complex processes which keep us alive and well each day. From discussing just these four, it is easier to understand how important our healthy diet really is. Sleep, of course, is important and taking measures to reduce stress in our lives. However, now you understand a little more about how to improve sleep and how to improve your body's tolerance and perception of stress.

Are you surprised to learn how much of our lives are influenced by our diet? Are you surprised to learn that simply eating more of certain foods can help us sleep more deeply, feel calmer, can improve our pain tolerance and even improve our focus and motivation?

I hope that you enjoyed this chapter, I did enjoy writing it for you. Now my dopamine sensors are firing up to provide me with the sense of achievement from having taken the time to help others. A free buzz I'm willing to happily accept.

Let's now talk about specific ways that we can reduce stress, without gorging on chocolate!

# Meditative Eating

As a Buddhist, I'm a big fan of Meditation, but I'll be honest, I'm not always good at it. I have a highly active brain which loves to problem solve, it hardly ever quietens down and often when I need it to be most peaceful it is at it's noisiest.

Meditation is something that has gained a lot of popularity recently, however far beyond a fad, this ancient practice has been used for thousands of years to connect with the earth / god / gods / buddhas / divine / universe etc.

In modern day society, we have a greater need for meditation than ever before. Many of our daily practices in previous decades were meditative, however, with the rise of technology, these are now becoming less common. Methods such as painting, knitting, reading, sewing, praying, gardening, crochet, pottery, cooking and eating, when done correctly can be considered meditative. Meditative practice is where we calmly focus on only one task for an extended period of time.

Even walking used to be a meditative task. We would take in our surroundings, drink in the sounds, the smells, the sights. Now we walk along hurriedly, usually with a smartphone in hand, checking emails, social media feeds, calling or texting someone or listening to music.

When was the last time you took a peaceful walk without your smartphone?The rise of technology has decreased our attention span and increased our stress levels. We rush everywhere now and are often multi-tasking. This increases stress and diminishes productivity. I challenge you this week to take a moment when you're next walking somewhere, ask yourself if you are rushing. If so, ask yourself if you really need to hurry. Is it more important to get to your destination quickly or calmly? Will the world be better or worse for you taking a few deep breaths, smelling the flowers, appreciating the sun on your face, enjoying the view, watching the birds etc?

## When did you last read a book cover to cover?

We can't even get through a book now without purchasing the next one mid-way through. Often we may be reading 2 to 5 books at any one time, we become bored quickly, overstimulated with inspiration for the next idea, the next topic. We literally cannot sit still.

In my opinion, this is one of the biggest pitfalls of an E-Book. I've always been a bigger fan of the real thing, however when people ask me why I could only say "It's the smell and feel of the paper" or "I don't know I just find real books much more calming".

It took me a little while, but I jumped on the Kindle bandwagon too. So many books at my fingertips. A bookworm's dream. However, it's my experience with E-books that have made me realise what it is about a real book that is so special.

Just the mere fact that you know you have literally hundreds of thousands of other books at your fingertips makes it really difficult to commit.  And kindle have made it even easier for us to be non-committal, by offering Kindle unlimited, "download a sample" and also by suggesting other books that are "mentioned in this book".

How are we supposed to lose ourselves in any one book when we have all of this temptation?

With a real-life book, you pick it up, read until you're bored, exhausted (or about to miss your stop). You get lost in the book. You may think of other books, it may stimulate ideas, it may even mention other books. You may take note to go to the bookstore and buy this other book. However, when it's immediately accessible, it's far too tempting and therefore difficult to maintain focus.

How many books are you currently reading in conjunction with this one? I challenge you to commit to just this book, even if only for this week. You'll find you'll relax more, will learn more and will find it much easier to regain that wonderful feeling of falling down the rabbit hole and losing yourself in the story. It's a really great feeling.

## When did you last eat alone, without touching your phone?

On your next lunch break, I challenge you to look around you. Everyone who sits alone will be on their phone. Mindlessly shovelling in mouthfuls of foods, often still stabbing away at the empty bowl and then wondering where it all went. This might remind you of someone. That someone might be you.

Eating, when done right, is an incredibly meditative process. Here's my 3 step guide to meditative eating:

## Step 1: Be thankful

Take a moment to appreciate the food in front of you. If you bought or made the meal yourself, then you chose this meal for a reason. Are there ingredients which you really enjoy? Are there ingredients which you know will enrich your health? Take a moment to recognise this bowl of medicine that you have in front of you. What are the benefits of this meal? Does it contain healing foods / high protein foods / healthy fats / healing herbs and spices? Be thankful for the ability to sit down and eat this meal at a time when you are hungry.

If you didn't make the meal yourself, be thankful to the person who did make it. Take a moment, as you appreciate the colours, the smells, the presentation of the meal, also to be thankful for the person who put this meal together for you. Did they choose your favourite? Did they add ingredients which will assist you with your health? Did they spend time experimenting with a new meal in a hope to impress you or make you happy?

## Step 2: Appreciate the flavours and textures

As you place the food in your mouth now, take a moment as you chew to really appreciate the flavours and textures of the food you are eating.

Enjoy the sensation of eating, the feeling of rewarding your body with nutrients which will improve your health. Every time we choose to eat, we choose to live. Enjoy this choice. Chew your food slowly and focus on each different flavour and texture within your meal.

## Step 3: Chew slowly

Chew your food slowly, until it forms a paste in your mouth. Breathe deeply and slowly as you eat. Don't rush or hurry, remind yourself that there is all the time in the world. The more time you allow yourself to take to eat your meals, the more nutrients you will gain from lesser quantities. This will lead to easier weight management, improved enjoyment of meals, improved energy, happiness and general health.

This practice, not only improves your appreciation for all foods, including really healthy ones, it also significantly enhances digestion. Digestion begins in the mouth, where we secrete digestive enzymes to break down starches and sugars. While chewing, each flavour and texture perceived signals to the brain of what specific enzymes and digestive processes will best assist in the breakdown of this food and absorption of nutrients. By taking the time to enjoy our meal, we improve our digestion, increase our absorption of nutrients and therefore improve the healing benefit of each meal.

# Meditation Apps

**M**editation apps are one of the best things to come out of modern technology. In an age where technology has significantly reduced our capacity to pay attention and has increased our stress levels, it has also come to the rescue for the very same problems.

As a Buddhist, I'm really supposed to be a purist. I'm probably supposed to scoff at the idea of a developer making millions of dollars from meditation subscriptions. However, I find meditation apps to be an incredibly valuable and helpful resource for both myself and my patients.

With 7 years of practice as a healthcare practitioner in Sydney's central business district, I've seen my share of overworked and highly stressed patients. In my consultations, I have introduced a 5-10 minute meditation segment for many of my patients. I either talk them through a body scan or use one of the meditation apps while the patient is lying down on the comfy, padded massage bed for me to take their body composition and cellular health reading.

For many of them, this is the only point in the day where they get to relax. I've had people walk in red-faced, twitching and on the verge of tears. These same people after 5-10 minutes of listening to a simple meditation, appear to float out of the clinic. They are calmer, happier and feeling more positive. Those few minutes can make all the difference.

I encourage almost all my patients to make use of meditation apps. These apps allow the benefits of meditation in a highly portable and user-friendly format. Just put on your headphones, close your eyes, and you're ready to go. No chanting, oms or mudras (hand gestures) required. Just close your eyes, place your hands on your knees and listen as they walk you through it.

Apps make the process incredibly simple and are a great way to decrease stress. New ones are popping up all the time. However, my two favourites are Headspace and Calm.

## Headspace

Headspace is excellent for even absolute beginners, sceptics, no-nonsense people and men who are not into "that airy fairy rubbish" - their words, not mine.

Headspace has a great "10 for 10" introductory course. Where you do 10 minutes of meditation every day for 10 days. It's a man's voice, speaking clearly and walking you through a straightforward and easy to follow process to clear your mind. There are a few animations along the way which help to explain what meditation really is, rather than what we perceive it to be in our over-thinking.

When you get through the 10 for 10 series, you can choose to upgrade to unlock the rest of the foundation pack. After 30 sessions within the foundation pack, you "graduate" to unlock other packs which can be specific to particular topics.

There is also a panic button. This is great for when you've had or have an uncomfortable discussion or presentation to give. This is a

3-minute meditation designed to bring you back to neutral quickly.

There are meditations to improve sleep, decrease stress, improve relationships, decrease pain and many more. In summary, Headspace is a great tool to have to help improve your health and wellbeing through a healthy mindset.

## Calm

Calm is my favourite for a few reasons: Firstly it has a female voice, which I find equally soothing and nurturing. Secondly, there are nature sounds which you can play in the background of your meditation. I find these very powerful for quickly increasing relaxation and actually have started playing these nature sounds when at work and in need of calming, better focus or increased creativity. If patients appear to be stressed I may also play nature sounds while we speak, to assist them with relaxing and opening up. Many go on to purchase the app as they find these sounds to be so soothing.

Thirdly, Calm has sleep stories. These are stories such as The Velveteen Rabbit, The Emperors New Clothes, plus nature essays, Shakespeare and many more. They are spoken in a soothing voice and designed specifically to improve relaxation and assist with deeper sleep. I find this feature incredibly beneficial and use this feature on most nights.

Calm also has "packs" or courses which are focused on particular topics. However, they also run "Daily Calm"s which are daily meditations with topics that may be relevant to the day of the week, key dates, holidays or current events.

Personally, in addition to my daily Buddhist chanting and reflection, I also try to do a "Daily Calm" each day, listen to the nature sounds while working and also listen to a sleep story most nights. I find this helps me stay grounded, focused, calmer and happier, even at the most stressful of times.

I would recommend that you take some time to experiment with meditation this week. Try incorporating a 10-minute meditation to your day.

# De-Stress With an Anti-Inflammatory Diet

Stress is a highly inflammatory state, which prevents healing, decreases sleep quality, inhibits digestion and increases energy expenditure. This leads to you feeling flat, fatigued, forgetful and malnourished in a matter of days.

Chronic stress, even at a low-grade or mild level, can significantly reduce your health and wellbeing.

For years many people have turned to antidepressants to assist with getting through a stressful period. In some cases people find the results to be favourable, however, what many people do not know is that these drugs are very addictive, physically, and coming off them is not a pleasant or quick process.

However, here's something interesting that has arisen in recent years. Antidepressants are now considered to be mostly useful due to their effects on decreasing inflammation, rather than the changes in the serotonin metabolism. This is incredible news as we have an insanely powerful anti-inflammatory medicine at our disposal - the anti-inflammatory diet.

The anti-inflammatory diet is one which is rich in green leafy vegetables, oily fish, olives, extra virgin olive oil, avocado, eggs, raw nuts and seeds, turmeric and fresh fruit.

This diet is also free of processed foods, refined carbohydrates, high sugar foods, gluten-containing grains, dairy products (except greek yoghurt and kefir), refined soy products. Caffeine and alcohol are to be kept to a minimum and from only natural sources.

This diet is highly nourishing, delicious, enjoyable and easy to follow. I'd even go so far as to say that it is the healthiest diet overall. Let's go through a few key points.

## Green leafy vegetables

Rich in anti-inflammatory vitamin k, vitamin E, calcium, potassium, magnesium, iron and folic acid (among others), green leafy vegetables are really a nutritional powerhouse and yet they contain the lowest number of calories (typically only about 25calories per cup). This means we can fill up on these green goodies and soak up all of their healing benefits with little concern for our daily calorie budget.

I recommend aiming to eat 2 cups (or 2 handfuls) of green vegetables with every meal. If greens don't go with the recipe (this is unusual) then just add a side salad of rocket and spinach with basil or fresh mint. Or even snack on a handful or two of rocket before eating. This also adds another benefit of improving digestion.

## Good Fats

Oily fish contains omega 3 fatty acids, which are our 'good fats'. These fats are essential for human life and help to reduce inflammation. The fats found in fish are called Eicosapentaenoic Acid (EPA) and Docosa-hexaenoic acid (DHA). In plant sources, we have Alpha Linolenic Acid (ALA) which our body then converts to the active form. EPA and DHA are much more potent anti-inflammatory agents than ALA and are considered the go-to in inflammatory conditions.

Oily fish such as salmon, sardines, mackerel and trout include higher concentrations of these therapeutic oils, in combination with higher amounts of Vitamins A and D.

Omega 3 fats are also vital for healthy metabolism, another therapeutic use during stress to combat the stress-induced belly bulge.

## Olives and Extra Virgin Olive Oil

Olives and Extra Virgin Olive Oil are to be used liberally in the anti-inflammatory diet. Olives contain a natural substance called oleocanthal which possesses similar anti-inflammatory properties to ibuprofen, without any of the adverse side effects typically seen with the drug.

Olives can be eaten as a snack, added to salads, included in omelettes or blended to form a dip for fresh raw vegetables. Extra virgin olive oil is best enjoyed as a dressing for salads. However, good quality, slightly alkaline olive oils are stable for up to 200degrees and therefore can be used in cooking.

Olives also contain valuable vitamin E and are effective in reducing blood cholesterol.

## Avocado

Avocados contain valuable vitamin E which decreases inflammation, is a powerful antioxidant and is said to be anti-aging.

Avocados are also an excellent source of dietary fibre and protein and many essential nutrients including B Vitamins, Vitamin D, Vitamin C, CoQ10 and many more. Mostly, they are known for being rich in healthy fats which reduce inflammation and promote healthy, youthful skin.

## Turmeric

Turmeric is an anti-inflammatory, antiviral, antibacterial and mood-boosting herb.

Studies have compared the effects of turmeric extract to Prozac. Prozac is a widely recognised, effective antidepressant which, like all others, is highly addictive and may result in many adverse side effects. In one particular study, the turmeric extract demonstrated only a 2% less impact than the antidepressant in improving energy, mood and motivation.

This same study also assessed the effects of turmeric when combined with Prozac and found the results to be even more effective than Prozac alone.

This is a powerful demonstration of the incredible resources and natural medicines which we have available to us at a low cost. Turmeric is widely available, highly therapeutic and should always be considered during times of stress.

## Three ways to get more turmeric into your day:

Try a turmeric latte or make a home-made turmeric and ginger tea. These beverages are surprisingly good, and many people notice immediate mood-boosting effects.

Mix a salad dressing of extra virgin olive oil, turmeric, lemon juice and, if you like, add a little ginger. This super anti-inflammatory elixir can be used to dress your salads, veggies or added to eggs to increase the flavour and healing properties of your meals.

· Make homemade veggie curries or dahl to consume as between-meal snacks or to serve with brown rice or quinoa. Be sure to add lots of turmeric, garlic and other relevant spices for that powerful anti-inflammatory boost.

# Week 5 Reflection

Now that you have taken time to reflect on the stressors in your life, and with your new found understanding of the physiological consequences of stress, how do you feel?

This week we've learned how stress negatively effects our life, what effects our diet and lifestyle choices can have on our emotions, and have discussed methods for reducing daily stress, through meditative eating and mindfulness.

Now it's time to reflect on this week's lessons. What did you find most interesting? What can you commit to in order to create a positive change and reduce the effects of stress on your life?

**Week 5 Checklist:**
1. What stressors do you have control over?
2. What measures can you implement to remove or reduce these stressors? (Remember to use the SMART goals system here)
3. What small changes can you make to your diet to enhance your stress resilience? (For example, could you drink more tea or eat daily fermented foods?)
4. What mindfulness practice would you be happy to commit to daily? Could you introduce mindful eating or a meditation app?

For those of you who are overwhelmed by stress, writing out your stressors and committing to change can feel even more overwhelming and at times completely unachievable. For this I have a suggested protocol.

- Day 1: Write out the stressors that you have control over (such as not getting enough sleep, over-committing yourself etc.)
- Day 2: In a calm environment (during the day so that it doesn't over excite you or prevent sleep) write out those stressors that you do not have control over. Sometimes identifying the gravity of your situation assists you to recognise when help is needed.
- Day 3: Write out the possible changes you could make to your diet and lifestyle. Include everything from "I'll stop putting so-and-so before my own needs" to "I'll drink less coffee and drink more tea". This is an empowering exercise which will help you to feel more in charge.
- Day 4: Commit to a schedule for change utilising SMART goals. Set Small, Measurable, Accountable, Realistic and Time Based goals such as "I will reduce my coffee by 1 cup each day, replacing each cup with tea."

# VIII

# Week 6: Building better energy

# Alkalise to Energise

So far we have addressed many major pillars of health. We've put in place a healthier, more balanced diet, have incorporated some therapeutic foods, have worked on improving sleep and last week we discussed some great stress-busting tactics. This week we're going to focus on our energy. By now hopefully, you're sleeping a little better, feeling a little less stressed and feeling confident in your dietary choices. I hope that you are enjoying your meals and feeling inspired and energised after eating them.

However, if you're recovering from, or currently undergoing, any major stress (emotional or physical) then your energy may still need a little extra help. Let's discuss this further.

One of my favourite dietary principles to teach is an acid-alkaline balance. Following this principle often offers substantial improvements in energy and vitality in a matter of days, particularly when combined with lots of anti-inflammatory foods.

Many of my patients have achieved goals they never thought possible by applying this approach. Even patients who come in with an excellent foundation diet notice substantial further improvements when they introduce the alkalising approach.

When provided with the information and tools and, due to the foods which are required to be consumed, consuming more alkalising foods simultaneously addresses many other health concerns by default.

This is taking the vegetable and therapeutic intake to the next level, not just eating more of them but using them to counterbalance many of the challenges of daily living.  Alkalising foods help to reduce post-prandial fatigue (that post-meal slump) and can substantially improve your energy with one simple dietary focus. You'll also notice that there's a bit of cross over from last week, as most alkalising foods are also anti-inflammatory. So, rather than beginning a whole new approach this week, we're simply building on a deeper understanding on how some of these therapeutic foods work, and how we can optimise/balance our intake for maximum effects.

## What are alkaline foods and why do we need them?...

We are alkaline by design, acidic by nature. What this means is our bodily functions require an alkaline pH, however many of our regular daily processes cause acidity. Our blood is a mildly alkaline substance with a pH of around 7.365

Note:  The pH scale runs 0-14, neutral is 7, the alkaline range is between 7-14, the acidic range is between 0-7.

It is absolutely vital that we maintain our mildly alkaline blood pH and our body will do everything possible to ensure this. We will use any available resource to stabilise the pH. This includes using calcium from bones or glutamine from muscles in times of desperate need.

Many of our daily processes, including digestion and tissue repair, elevate acidity. Some factors substantially increase acidity, such as stress, sickness and toxicity. Yes that includes recovering from a few glasses of vino.

If our diet does not supply adequate amounts of alkalising nutrients, our resources begin to run low. If we then become unwell, stressed or injured, then we will need to deplete these valuable reserves in our bones and muscles.

You have probably felt the effects of acidity, without even knowing it. The reason we feel sore and achy as if we've run a marathon after the flu is because we have shredded muscle tissue to release glutamine in a desperate attempt to alkalise the blood. This can also happen during times of severe or chronic stress, which again leads to aches and pains.

So how do we counteract this? Do we need to take alkalising supplements? Do we need to take supplemental glutamine?

The answer is simple. In most cases, all we need to do is to eat a diet rich in foods which contain alkalising nutrients and to ensure that any time we consume acidic foods, we balance them with alkalising foods.

If we are particularly sick, toxic, stressed or injured, then supplements can really help to get us more quickly back on track. However, the long-term approach is to maintain an optimal intake of alkalising foods.

Note: If your aim is to merely prevent sickness then you can achieve this by just ensuring you have 2-3 cups of vegetables each day. If however, you want to reach the highest level of health and vitality, I recommend eating more alkaline foods.

By balancing the acid-alkaline foods within your meals, you will find that you experience a more significant energy boost from each meal. You'll begin to wake with more energy, and it will be more consistent throughout the day. You may also find that you sleep much more deeply as an alkaline body performs and repairs much more efficiently, leading to less energy wastage at all times, even at rest.

If you follow a diet rich in alkalising foods, while also being sure to include adequate protein and fats of course (more on this soon), then you'll become superhuman. You'll experience a higher level of energy and vitality, you'll be in better shape, better health and with a better state of mind.

Many people live on acidic diets, with high stress for many years which leads to extreme fatigue and can increase the feeling of hopelessness and lack of motivation to change. It is tough to take on the challenge of change while you are feeling physically and emotionally weak. Trust me, I've been there!

## Acid-Alkaline Balance

Let me give you a couple of examples of meals and how we can modify them to supercharge their effects.

First let's say you have a cheese omelette for breakfast, with a slice of rye toast and a side of black tea/coffee/orange juice. These are all acidic foods. Therefore even if your eggs, cheese, bread and beverage were made from organic, healthy ingredients, the fact that your meal is not well balanced might lead to you feeling drained, over-full and possibly suffering from heartburn.

Now let's switch it up and include some alkalising foods. Let's say we had a spinach omelette with just a little cheese (or no cheese), a side of avocado and carbohydrates were potato, sweet potato, brown rice or quinoa (alkalising carbohydrate sources). For a drink, rather than black tea or coffee, you had a glass of water with fresh lemon juice. This would now be an alkalising meal.

This is how this works:

- Acidic foods: Eggs, Cheese, Tea/Coffee/Juice, Bread
- Alkalising foods: Lemon, Spinach, Avocado,

Pair one acid food (egg) with one alkalising food (spinach) for a balanced meal. Add in more alkalising foods (avocado and lemon), and you have an alkaline meal which will stock up your mineral reserves. You'll also be reducing the need to expend energy alkalising from the digestion of acidic foods and will feel lighter and more energetic as a result.

When discussing the example of the cheese omelette with my patients, many can affiliate with the fatigued feeling that results. Those same patients notice a significant improvement when taking the time to prepare balanced or alkaline meals and report feeling a noticeable improvement in their overall energy and general wellbeing.

## Alkalising foods - The cheat sheet to healthy eating?

We could consider alkalising foods as a cheat sheet for healthy eating. Not only are these foods rich in minerals and decrease the need to deplete valuable nutrients, but they are also incredibly healthy foods and do not include any unhealthy foods at all.

## Benefits of an alkalising diet:

- Rich in plant-based, natural foods
- Restricts high-sugar and processed foods
- Encourages consumption of low-GI, fibre rich foods

- Discourages use of caffeinated beverages and soft drinks
- Rich in vegetables and fruits which provide essential vitamins, minerals and antioxidants

## The disadvantage of an alkalising diet:

If misunderstood, may discourage the intake of protein-rich foods such as fish, meats, eggs etc.

## How to eat daily

A daily intake rich in alkalising foods would look something like this:
- On rising - drink a glass of water with fresh lemon or lime
- Breakfast - Spinach omelette with avocado OR Purple Power Smoothie (see recipes)
- Snack - Celery, Carrot, capsicum and Cucumber sticks dipped in tahini or almond butter
- Lunch - 3 handfuls of fresh veggies, rich in greens, a half cup of beetroot, a palm-sized serve of protein, fresh lemon juice, extra virgin olive oil.
- Snack - green smoothie
- Dinner - 3 handfuls of fresh veggies, rich in greens, a palm-sized serve of protein, half a cup of quinoa, tahini and lemon juice dressing

## Alkaline diet cheat sheet

- All vegetables are alkalising. Spinach, Kale, Kelp, Broccoli and Sprouts are Highly alkalising.
- Fruits: Lemon, Lime, Grapefruit, Coconut are alkalising. Rock-melon (cantaloupe), dried fruits, Nectarines, Plum, Watermelon

and Cherries are Neutral. All other fruits are acidic (yet still very healthy).

- Grains and Pulses: All beans (such as Butterbeans, Soybeans, Haricot beans, Black beans etc.) Quinoa, Spelt, Buckwheat, Lentils and tofu are alkalising. Amaranth, Oats, Millet and Spelt are neutral. All other grains are acidic.
- Protein sources: Tofu, Lentils and Beans mentioned above, Goat milk and goats yoghurt are alkalising. Freshwater wild fish and protein powders made from brown rice, hemp or pea protein are neutral. All meats, fish, eggs and cow's milk dairy products are acidic.
- Nuts and seeds: Chia seeds, sesame seeds and almonds soaked in water are alkaline. Brazil, Pecan, Hazelnuts and Walnuts are neutral. All other nuts and seeds are acidic.

# Audit the "Energy Leak"

When trying to improve our energy, it's important that we also take time to reduce those factors which are currently draining our reserves and demanding more energy than they should. Inevitably there will be some that we have no control over, such as taking care of young children. However, there are often other factors which we can control.

Think of this like saving money on your electricity bill. There's no point switching to the cheapest provider and then leaving the lights on all day long. For this reason, this week's content is also a little lighter. Allowing you more time to reflect and modify, with less required reading time.

Below is a list of factors which we can address to reduce the daily "energy leak". Take a look and see what changes you can commit to making. Check an item off the list each time you have addressed it to create a sense of achievement and empowerment.

- Improve the quality and duration of your sleep. We discussed lots of ways to do this last week.
- Prioritise your own needs and start saying no to commitments that are not either fun or necessary. This is not easy initially, but it gets easier over time.
- Set standardised work hours and do not allow yourself to check emails, your to-do list or your schedule for your week outside of these hours. This preserves your "me time" for recharging and

relaxing and will lead to a more productive, less stressed week ahead.

- Take time out for fun and relaxation every day. I recommend 30 minutes each and every day. Set an alarm for this with a fun tone. This can be 30 minutes of dancing around your living room to your favourite music, walking in green space, yoga, reading, researching, drawing, painting, playing fetch with your pet or hide and seek with your little ones, whatever fills you up.
- Remove unnecessary chemical stressors, eat organic or wash your fruits and veggies, use natural skin care and cleaning products etc. (Tip: We'll address this further in week 8)
- Reduce your coffee and sugar intake and rely on natural energisers like alkaline foods. You'll be surprised at the improvements in your skin, mood, sleep, and ultimately your energy. Coffee consumption makes us feel that it's giving us energy, when in fact it's just forcing us to produce it more quickly, using up all of your vital nutrients along the way.

# Hydrate, Hydrate, Hydrate

I am often surprised at how many patients come to me having already made significant improvements to their diet and yet still missing one of the most vital pieces of the puzzle.

Many people increase their vegetable intake, reduce their portion size, reduce processed foods, take a probiotic, take a multivitamin, increase their exercise etc.. And yet they are drinking no more than 1L of water per day.

So few people seem to comprehend the importance of optimal hydration, or how to achieve it. It's quite shocking.

So let's discuss this important issue right now and, please, make me a promise that you will address this and make it your primary focal point.

## Hydration

What does it mean to have proper hydration? Does it mean drinking 2L each day? Is this enough? Does it matter what gender you are? Does your frame size matter? Does your exercise activity impact your requirements? Does it matter what you drink?

Let's discuss each of these points in detail now to ensure there is no confusion.

## Is 2L of water per day enough?

2 litres of water per day may or may not be enough for you. The 2-litre guideline is set as a recommended average. However, where you live, the conditions and nature of your work, your frame size, your gender and your dietary choices will all impact your fluid requirements.

If you are a female of around 5'6 or below, you work and live in a moderate climate with no extreme temperatures, you eat a healthy diet and have no pre-existing conditions, then 2 litres is enough for you. However on days that you exercise this minimum requirement is going to increase.

## What does it mean to have proper hydration?

Proper hydration means that you have an adequate supply of fluids to keep all organs and tissues hydrated. It means that there is water inside the cells which keeps them healthy and plump (think grapes). It means that there are enough electrolytes to hold the water inside the cells (we'll discuss electrolytes in a moment). It means that there is enough fluid to regularly flush the kidneys, bladder and urinary tract which keeps them healthy. It also means that there is enough to keep your poop nice and soft and easy to pass.

Being well hydrated allows your body to flush and eliminate toxins. You remove water and fat-soluble toxins from the body through your urine, stools and perspiration. When you are well hydrated, these elimination pathways work quickly and efficiently, keeping you healthy and protected. When you are dehydrated these pathways slow down, leading to a decreased ability to detox which leads to toxic buildup. You feel stressed, fatigued, grumpy and may experience physical side effects such as headaches, muscle weakness or weight gain.

## How do I figure out how much I need?

Firstly, your gender plays a big part in determining your ideal water intake. As muscle cells carry a significant amount of water, the more muscle you have, the more water you require. Women usually carry a higher body fat percentage than men. Women are at our healthiest at between 20-27% body fat. Men, however, have an ideal range of 10-17%.

To calculate your baseline water needs multiply your weight in kilos by 28. This will give you the volume in millilitres that you need to consume. If you are male, I recommend multiplying this number by 1.5. The higher muscle percentage of a male requires a higher fluid intake.

Next, it's time to determine how much you need on an exercise day. There are two ways to calculate this. Option 1 is to just drink an extra 350ml for every half an hour you exercise. This is the standard recommendation.

However, we all know that half an hour of gentle walking gets you much less sweaty than half an hour of high-intensity interval training or running. Therefore it's easy to understand that different forms of exercise require different re-hydration strategies.

If you would like to calculate your specific needs, there is a simple home-test. Before beginning your exercise routine, stand on the scale (preferably without clothes). Drink an exact amount during your session. This can be anything from 250ml to 1L, but it needs to be precise as you will need it for your calculation.

After your workout, strip off your sweaty clothes and towel off as much as possible, now weigh yourself again. If you weigh 1kg less then you have sweat out roughly 1L of water. If you drank 500ml during the session, then you have actually lost that too. So your total sweat volume for this exercise intensity and duration is 1.5L. This means that on a day that you perform this activity you must drink your baseline amount, plus the 1.5L extra.

## How do we achieve proper hydration?

As we've just discussed, there are many factors which need to be considered when determining your ideal fluid intake. We have reviewed the need to factor in our gender, weight, activity duration and intensity when determining our specific needs.

A critical consideration and an essential rule for improving your hydration is your diet. A healthy balanced diet which is rich in fresh vegetables and fruits will contribute towards your total water requirements.

More than just the water they contain, fresh fruits and vegetables contribute electrolytes, support the kidneys and promote regular elimination of wastes through the bowel.

Some foods are more hydrating than others. Celery, cucumber, watermelon and iceberg lettuce have high water content and provide necessary minerals to support kidney health.

Swapping processed foods with healthy, plant-based, natural food sources will improve your hydration significantly. Even trading your grains for a side of potato, sweet potato, pumpkin and zucchini can provide considerably more water.

Consuming refined sugar and poorly controlled blood sugar is highly taxing on the kidneys and can lead to excessive thirst coupled with water retention. The kidneys are a powerful filter system which can become easily damaged when they are overused. High sugar intake, high protein intake and high alcohol intake lead to increased toxic wastes in the blood which places increased demand on the kidneys leading to damage, destruction and failure.

Vegetables help to support the kidneys, control blood sugar and promote elimination of wastes through the bowel. This decreases the load on our sensitive and invaluable kidneys. By increasing vegetables, decreasing processed foods, controlling our blood sugar and minimising exposure to alcohol, we keep the kidneys healthy.

Note: A high protein intake can result in increased toxic wastes in the blood leading to increased demand on the kidneys. Many cases of toxicity and kidney damage have been seen when a high protein diet is not followed correctly. This is why vegetables are important and why they are a crucial part of any higher protein diet.

Personally, I believe that a moderate protein, high vegetable diet is the more effective and safer choice. This approach offers significantly higher delivery of essential nutrients and fibre resulting in quick improvement in energy, vitality, mood, immunity and with equal, if not improved weight loss success. This approach also supports daily detoxification leading to better overall health in the long term, while also promoting the health of the kidneys and other vital organs.

## Caffeine, Coffee and Cola

Caffeinated drinks such as coffee, tea and cola are known as diuretics. This means that they increase the rate of fluid loss. You may have noticed that after too many coffees (for most people this is after just 1) it becomes difficult to hold your urine for more than 30-60 minutes. You feel like you are always on the toilet and the volume, colour and smell of your urine may even change.

It's not particularly difficult to understand that, if the rate of fluid loss has increased, your fluid requirements have too.

Cutting back on caffeinated beverages offers a host of health benefits.  Keeping with the topic at hand, cutting back on caffeine dramatically decreases your fluid loss, leading to better hydration and therefore better health and energy.  Try cutting down on your coffee and tea consumption. Ideal amounts are 1 coffee per day, 2-3 cups of green tea or 2 cups of black tea.

Note: Most herbal teas are caffeine free and contribute to your total fluid intake. Nettle tea is rich in electrolytes and good for the kidneys making this an excellent choice. Some herbal teas such as dandelion are diuretic and therefore should be consumed in moderation.

Sugary caffeinated beverages such as energy drinks, cola and even Mountain Dew (higher caffeine content than coke) double the hit on your hydration levels as they are both diuretic and high sugar. Replace your soft drinks with sparkling water and fresh lemon or lime juice.

## Additional considerations

If you are suffering from chronic kidney disease, or are currently pregnant or breastfeeding your fluid requirements may dramatically change. It is best to discuss your specific needs with your healthcare practitioner.

## Top 5 Tips for Improving Hydration

1. Start your day with a glass of water with fresh lemon or lime juice. These fruits are low sugar, rich in alkalising minerals and

contain electrolytes for improved absorption.

2. Eat the minimum 6 handfuls of fresh, raw vegetables every day. Particularly hydrating vegetables are cucumber, celery, iceberg lettuce, zucchini.

3. Snack on 1-2 pieces of fresh fruit each day. This does not include the lemon or lime you add to your water. Particularly hydrating fruits are watermelon, apples and citrus fruits.

4. Reduce caffeinated and sugary beverages which increase water loss. Swap soft drinks for sparkling water with fresh lemon or lime juice. Swap coffee for herbal tea or hot water with lemon.

5. Carry a water bottle with you everywhere you go. Drink a minimum of 2L per day if you are female, 2.5L if you are male. For best results, drink slowly in sips rather than guzzling at once.

# Keep Your Blood Sugar Stable

A healthy balanced diet can improve your energy, mood and general health in a matter of days. One of the most important rules about human nutrition is understanding how food affects your blood sugar. Concerningly, this is also one of the areas that I find most people know the least.

## What does it mean to control your blood sugar?

In the morning, when we wake, after a long fast, our blood sugar is typically quite low, usually at a level of around 4.5-5 when we are healthy (and haven't overeaten the night before). In an attempt to raise blood sugar, your body will send you the signal that you know as hunger, driving you to eat.

When we eat, the sugar glucose is released into our bloodstream. The amount of fibre, protein and fat in any particular meal has an effect on the rate at which those sugars are released.

Let's say that our baseline blood sugar has a number of zero. When our blood sugar elevates from zero, this signals the production of insulin by an organ called the pancreas. Insulin is the key that unlocks the gate of each cell, allowing glucose to travel through to be converted into energy inside a little cellular 'battery' called the Mitochondria.

The Mighty Mitochondria inside our cells are largely responsible for your energy and motivation. They are quick and efficient when appropriately nourished, but they require a plethora of nutrients to do their job. When we run low in these nutrients, our mitochondria can't turn our food into energy. This results in us feeling generally tired and lethargic, but will also result in other symptoms too. After all, the mitochondria don't just produce the energy we feel, but also the energy to keep vital organs and systems running. When they fail, systems fail, and we become unwell.

## What happens to the excess

It is normal for us to eat excess occasionally and our bodies are well equipped to deal with this. If your meal has provided more food (carbs, glucose, fats, or proteins) than you can absorb at any one time, it is considered excess and insulin will carry out its other duty which is to convert this excess to our backup or storage energy reserve (body fat).

To put it simply, we can say that when all is working well the process is as follows: We eat -> Blood sugar elevates -> The pancreas delivers insulin -> insulin unlocks the gates, opening up the channels so that food (glucose, fats and proteins) can flood in to the Mitochondria of the cell -> Cells create energy from food in the mitochondria -> Organs and systems run well -> We feel more energetic and motivated -> Any excess converts to body fat -> we feel full and stop eating.

However, this system works against us if we regularly overeat, if we overload our systems with too much glucose too quickly, or if our pancreas becomes exhausted and stops producing insulin. This is called diabetes type 1, the treatment is insulin injections.

When we are low in nutrients, the Mitochondria are slow in converting food to energy, resulting in a delayed absorption. This is perceived as excess, and we all know where the excess goes (your booty if you're lucky, your tummy if you're not). So the result is lower energy plus weight gain. If this happens over a longer period, the body tries to correct the balance by producing more insulin, yet the cells don't respond. This is diabetes type 2, or insulin resistance, which is a common result of an unhealthy diet, which is high in simple sugars and processed foods and low in nutrients.

What many people don't realise is that insulin resistance can be caused by stress. With your greater understanding of the process you should now be able to grasp why. Remember stress is "The Great Undoer" that drains our nutrient reserves and reduces our ability to absorb. With the nutrient deficiencies and increased demand, coupled with the unhealthy eating habits of stressful times, this often leads to insulin resistance, fatigue and weight gain. Yet another reason why eating a healthy balanced diet, and making lifestyle changes to address stress is so important.

## Balance your meals for optimum blood sugar control:

- **Eat high fibre carbs:** Fibre slows the release of sugar from foods. The more fibre your meal contains, the slower you will receive the sugar from foods and the more likely you'll respond with the exact amount of insulin your body needs to absorb the sugar. Prioritise your high fibre carbohydrates such as brown rice and legumes.
- **Eat protein in every meal**: Protein slows the release of sugar from foods. Protein is not broken down until it reaches the small intestine, unlike carbohydrates which break down in the mouth. This means, by adding in protein to your meals, when the carbs are all used up, you'll now produce energy from protein and amino acids. This is why protein-rich foods keep you full for longer.
- **Eat healthy fats:** Fats are taken into the blood around 3 hours after eating and remaining for up to 6 hours. Some fats are anti-inflammatory. Eat lots of these types of fats. As a supplement,

you may choose to take fish oil.

- **Eat alkalising foods:** Alkaline foods are rich in many of the vitamins and minerals responsible for converting "food" into energy. They are also high in antioxidants which helps to preserve and protect your mitochondria.

**Eat a variety of colours:** Each brightly coloured food has its own unique nutritional balance. Many of the colours have unique cell-preserving properties and play a vital role in protecting your mitochondria. Some brightly coloured foods are also protective of the pancreas such as sweet potato, red onions, turmeric and broccoli. What's more, seeing the variety on your plate is naturally stimulating and energising. This results in you feeling brighter, happier and more motivated.

# Week 6 Reflection

This week we took time to discuss how we can improve our energy through simple dietary and lifestyle changes. How do you feel after reviewing this information?

To help promote maximum energy, for you to live your happiest, healthiest life, let's set some SMART goals for the changes that will help.

Week 6 checklist

- Have you started incorporating more alkalising foods, or trying to better balance your meals?
- Have you audited the Energy-Leak in your life (those factors which deplete you)?
- Are you drinking more water each day?
- Are you balancing your meals to keep your blood sugar stable?
- Which of the above is most important for you? Which do you feel most able to work on?

Once you have answered the above questions you should be able to set yourself some SMART goals for building better energy. Next week we're going to work on putting that extra energy to good use with fun activities and exercise.

# IX

# Week 7: Your guide to exercise

# Do I Need to Exercise?

**N**ow that we've corrected a few fundamentals of a healthy, happy life and have worked on our energy levels, you should be waking up feeling more positive and ready for your day. With all this extra energy to burn, it's time to put it to good use and get moving. Let's talk about exercise.

Exercise is a key and fundamental component of any healthy living program. There are many processes in our bodies which rely on exercise for their stimulation. In short, exercise and movement are not optional. However, we certainly do have more choice than experts would like us to believe when it comes to the amount and types of exercise we are required to engage in.

## Why is exercise necessary?

Exercise helps to stimulate the improved growth of your mitochondria (the little batteries inside your cell where we produce energy from carbs, fats and proteins). The more we exercise, the more mitochondria we generate and, if we couple this with proper Nutrition, we also benefit from more efficient mitochondria. Remember these are the guys responsible for the energy you feel, and the energy required for organs and systems to function well and keep you healthy.

Exercise also assists with promoting natural detoxification which helps us to remove unnecessary wastes from the body. When we exercise we sweat which carries water-soluble toxins out through the skin's pores. The skin is our largest and, often, most under-utilised detoxification organ.

When we move, we also stimulate our internal detox drainage system, called the lymphatics. This system is not stimulated automatically, as the circulation is, but by movement alone. By exercising we improve the efficiency of this system and benefit from clearer skin, improved energy and easier weight loss.

The digestive system is also stimulated by physical movement. When we move, we engage the abdominal muscles, this stimulates the intestines, which helps to promote digestion and elimination. In return, we benefit from regular, more comfortable bowel movements, healthy, balanced appetite and easier weight management.

## Do I need to exercise?

We all need to exercise. That's not to say that we must be killing ourselves at the gym daily or running several kilometres per week. Exercise comes in many forms. However, we must all continue to move regularly to maintain a healthy happy body and mind.

You'll have seen an example of this in your older relatives. Those who stay active live longer, those who don't, unfortunately, deteriorate quickly, losing their energy, cognition, happiness and their desire to continue living. It's very sad to see. Try to keep the old ones around you as active as possible for as long as possible. Once they begin to slow down, it's very hard to get them going again.

However the same does ring true for us, it's just that it is much easier to reverse in us young folk. Taking time out to get moving each day keeps us young, flexible, strong, happy and healthy.

When we're feeling blue, it's often hard to get moving. I am one of the worst for this. During stressful times I could spend days at home reading, watching tv, flicking through social media etc. rather than actually getting out and participating in the world. This is my physiological response to my developmental years, my cortisol receptors burned out and as an adult stress now makes me physically exhausted. An interesting fact is that when there are high levels of cortisol in conjunction with high levels of sugar, the cortisol receptors seem to withstand greater levels of stress in the short term. Maybe this is the reason that many of us retreat to the couch, covered with a cozy blanket, comforted by junk food and TV when we're feeling hurt, depressed or unhappy.

However, one of the best ways to take charge of your health and happiness, reset the stress hormones and start enjoying life again is to move our body's. Exercise rebalances stress hormones, improves endorphin release and, quite honestly, there's nothing like feeling physically strong for improving your emotional strength. Changes can be significant and can happen within hours.

It is for this exact reason that a few years ago I ran a meetup group called FitFunFemales. I wanted to help women to get out and get active, to make new healthy friendships through healthy activities. I organised paddle boarding, long walks outdoors followed by healthy lunches, yoga in the park, and really anything else I could think of. It was great fun while I had the time and I met a lot of great people along the way.

If you're not interested in traditional exercise programs and would like to do fun outdoor activities, or you just would like to meet more people with similar interests, I highly recommend www.meetup.com.

Interestingly it's exercise that kick-started 21 year old Jen's journey to changing her life. After joining a gym and going regularly, 21 yr old Jen began feeling energised, enjoying life a little more and feeling stronger and more resilient. As her physical strength regained, she felt emotionally strong too. She started considering what life could look like if she made some changes, maybe even got out of that house. In the end, it was physical fitness that saved her life. Not because she could fight back, but because she could outrun. But we'll come back to that later...

# What Type of Exercise Should I Do?

Often people tell me that they don't have the time, energy or they just really struggle with the motivation to exercise. However, most of these same people know that exercise WILL help them feel better, eat better, sleep better, reduce their anxiety etc. Despite knowing this, however, it seems that the idea of trying to fit in an hour of hard slog a few times per week, regardless of the benefits, is just a daunting task that is too hard to implement.

I believe one of the reasons we have such a fear of adding in exercise to an already overstuffed schedule is that we've made it all so serious! Like if it's not the latest and most fashionable workout, then you're wasting your time.

I've heard all kinds of crazy things. It doesn't work unless it's HIIT, powerlifting, ultra-endurance, functional training etc. etc. etc.

The truth is that ALL exercise which raises the heart rate and gets you sweating is valuable and worthwhile. Anything that challenges you physically and mentally is worthwhile. Anything that stops you stressing about your work/bills/relationship etc. (even if only for half an hour) is worthwhile!

There are lots of fabulous exercise types out there, from exercises you do alone at home, to those you do as a group or a team. You could run outdoors, run on a treadmill, do resistance weight training, do yoga outdoors, in a gym or at a blissful yoga studio. You could join a basketball team, hockey team or do swim squad training.

There is an activity which suits every personality, every budget and every health condition. While there are lots of new and exciting forms of exercise which show promising results in research and studies. There really isn't a more perfect form of exercise than the one that gets you out of bed in the morning, off the couch on a Saturday, or to leave work on time through the week. The exercise that excites you is almost always the best.

Here are a few fun facts about exercise:

- Whatever you do, if you sweat for an hour you're eliminating toxins.
- If you're challenging your muscles and creating resistance, you're encouraging growth and regeneration of the muscles and bones.
- If your heart rate is up, you're burning calories and improving your lung capacity and heart health.
- If you reduce your stress response and calm enough so that you can sleep and feel more balanced, then you are reducing your chances of many chronic diseases.
- If you are doing movements which challenge coordination such as basketball, dance class etc. then you are rebuilding pathways in the brain that may lead to better creativity and focus in all areas of life (and better coordination for less falls in later life).

No matter what, in my mind, the fun is the most crucial part, particularly when you're stressed or depressed. How often do you lose yourself in something beneficial? How often do you let your hair down while sober? How often do you do something that takes you back to the here and now with an all-out sweat session that leaves you exhilarated?

We need to do more things that require sweat, fun, tears and total focus.  More of this leaves you feeling balanced, happy, motivated and less stressed, while also offering the increased calorie burning, muscle growth, increased energy and fitness etc. plus of course better sleep.

As you can see, there are benefits to most types of exercise. Just find something that gets you excited and do it often. It doesn't matter if it's fashionable / cool / sexy etc. It doesn't matter if it's Instagram worthy (you should see me at the end of a workout. I'm a red-faced sweat monster). Find something that gets you moving, get that heart rate up, get your sweat on. Find something fun, something that you can look forward to.

In summary:  Get your butt moving in the most fun way possible. Exercise with friends if they are up for it, join a meetup group, join a dance class, join a soccer or basketball team.

Whatever gets you sweaty and tired and laughing and excited all at the same time is excellent. Just get moving!

## Here are some ideas:

- Go paddle boarding or kayaking on the harbour with friends
- Join a dance class
- Join a basketball training group like this one
- Join a running group
- Do Zumba or try Pound
- Go to spin class
- Join an outrigger team
- Join a dragon boating team
- Try Lyra or Trampolining
- Try skipping, cartwheels or handstands

- Join an amateur soccer team
- Dance around your living room to your favourite music

Whatever it is, do what excites you, and you're much more likely to do it often. After all, there are very few, unhealthy, unfit athletes, no matter which sport they chose. The fact that they exercise frequently and passionately is all that matters.

There are also some great online resources for when you'd prefer a low-cost option or just to exercise at home. My preferred options are www.doyogawithme.com (a library of free yoga videos, something to suit every need) and www.bodyboss.com (a low-cost, home-based HIIT program with a gradual progression to suit all levels).

Choose what best suits you but commit to introducing more movement into your life, even if this is initially just more walking, yin yoga or light stretching.

# How Often Should I Exercise?

Ideally, we should do some sort of exercise daily. However, a minimum of 3 x per week is essential. If you're currently struggling to get a good exercise routine started, I'd recommend trying the day on day off rule.

## The Day on Day off Rule

Often new exercise habits are difficult to form. Usually, we start the week well, beginning with some hard, well-intentioned exercise. However the next day we wake up sore, maybe giving ourselves a few too many days to recover and before we know it the week is over.

An excellent way to get your exercise habit off to a great start is to set specific intentions. Rather than saying "I will exercise 3 x this week", tell yourself that you will exercise every second day. This method works best if you allow yourself to accumulate exercise days, i.e. exercise more than 1 day in a row, but you do not let yourself have more than 1 day off. If you follow this method, you'll find that you'll be exercising at least 3 x per week in no time. Many people see themselves exercising 4 or 5 days minimum using this method.

You see what tends to happen is that you wake up on Monday, you exercise, you feel great. This also means that you get to take tomorrow off. Then you wake up on Tuesday and realise you actually still feel pretty great, and if you exercise today then you get to take tomorrow off.  By Thursday you're usually exercising for your 3rd or 4th time already. You haven't taken more than 1 day off between sessions which means you've kept the momentum going.  You are getting progressively stronger, and fitter and developing a positive association with the way exercise makes you feel. Before you know it, you'll be exercising daily with enthusiasm.

# Eating for Exercise

I'd like to address the critical issue of eating for exercise. A common complication which I see in my practice is that when people begin exercising more, their appetite increases concomitantly. As we typically eat according to hunger, or for fear of being hungry, this usually results in weight gain.

Many people attend my practice stating that they are frequently exercising and eating well and just don't seem to be able to lose weight. In fact, some actually gain weight as a result. This is merely the result of eating incorrectly.

So now let's discuss three of the most common misconceptions and fundamentals of eating for exercise:

Can you exercise on an empty stomach?
What foods should you eat after exercise?
Do you need to carb load?
Do you need to eat more if exercising more?

## 1: Can you exercise on an empty stomach?

In short, yes. We all have adequate fuel in our bodies to exercise at moderate to high intensity for up to 1 and a half hours without eating anything prior or during. We are all equipped to get up from bed, stretch a little and then run for a full 90 minutes with no food in our stomachs. This is thanks to a carbohydrate fuel source called glycogen which we have in every muscle in the body.

This fuel source powers us up for a day of mild intensity activity or a couple of hours of moderate to high intensity. However, it must be replenished, once used, through the diet.

After we've exercised, we have a window of opportunity for optimum re-fuelling. This window is primarily due to an enzyme called glycogen synthase which takes carbohydrates and converts them to glycogen. Glycogen synthase is at it's highest for 1-2 hours after exercise. However, after 2 hours, the activity of this enzyme has mostly declined. Therefore it's essential to refuel with the appropriate food types shortly after exercise, to take advantage of this window of opportunity. Should you miss it, you're likely to feel tired and to be craving carbohydrates and/or sugar for the next 24hours, as your body desperately tries to recuperate glycogen, often reasonably unsuccessfully.

## 2: What foods should you eat after exercise?

Different forms of exercise, require different recovery meals. A recovery meal is the first meal consumed after a significant exercise session. Getting this meal right is the key to a quick recovery and looking forward to the next session.

There are a couple of rules when structuring your recovery meal. If you have performed an intense cardiovascular workout, then the general rule is to consume 1g of carbohydrates per kilogram of body weight, with a quarter to a third of this amount in protein.

For example, if you are a female who weighs 60kgs, you should consume 60g of carbohydrates. If you are trying to lose weight, then you should consume 20g of protein. This is the equivalent of 2.5 eggs and 2 large bananas, the perfect banana pancake mix. If however you are not trying to lose weight and are trying to fuel up quickly so that you can go out and exercise again later that day or the day following, then the protein content of this meal should be just 15g.

The ratio of carbohydrates to protein significantly affects the absorption. It is therefore vital to get this formula right.

If you have performed exercise that is mostly resistance work, a ratio of just 2:1 carbohydrates is sufficient. If you are a 60kg female who has completed a 45-minute weight training session, you should consume 60g of carbs and 30g of protein.

## 3: Do you need to carb load?

Carb loading is based on the theory that the more carbohydrates we eat, the more energised our muscles are as they are packed with glycogen (the carbohydrate fuel pack which we have in each muscle). However, carb loading is only appropriate to a point, and only for specific activities.

Mostly, carb loading is an inappropriate practice which contributes to weight gain, which can actually slow you down and inhibit performance more than contribute.

So when is carb loading appropriate? If you are about to run a half to full marathon, then this is a necessary practice which can have a significant impact on performance. However, if you are preparing to attend a gym session, perform a resistance based activity such as weight training, then carb loading is unnecessary and can result in weight gain.

## 4: Do I need to eat more if exercising more?

When you exercise, you burn nutrients, calories, protein and carbohydrates. These are nutrients which need to be replaced. However, it is important to remember that we are designed to be moving all day long, our body is well equipped to deal with significant volumes of movement each day, in short, a certain amount of activity is not just tolerated, it is expected.

Your body will crave more nutrients, and you will feel hungrier. However what you're mostly craving is nutrients, not calories, carbs or protein.  If you fuel your body wisely, you can improve your performance, recovery and energy while also losing any excess body weight or body fat.  If you do not change to a more nutritious diet, however, you'll find yourself insatiably hungry, tired and struggle to keep up the exercise.

# Revisiting SMART Goals

SMART goals are:

S : Specific, to ensure focus
M: Measurable, to ensure you are progressing
A: Agreed upon, to assure you are accountable
R: Realistic, to ensure you are capable of success
T: Time-based: In this case, 1 week each

Use this principle to map out some exercise goals that will be achievable. This is important for all health improvements, however, it feels particularly fitting to discuss it this week concerning exercise.

What would you like your life to be like in week 8? How do you want to feel? What would your new normal look like?

Use the SMART goals acronym to ensure that your intentions are specific, measurable, accountable, realistic and time-based. Doing so will significantly improve your ability to succeed.

# Week 7 Reflection

This week we have discussed how to incorporate exercise for maximum energy, health and happiness.

We've discussed how to choose the type of exercise which best suits you, how often we should exercise and how to eat for best results.

Finally we reviewed SMART goals, which is particularly important when starting out on a new regime. For those who are recovering from major health issues, stress or trauma, please promise me that you'll be kind to yourself and set yourself SMARKT goals (yes I just made that up). SMARKT stands for Small, Measurable, Agreed upon, Realistic, Kind and Time Measured. The idea here is that each goal helps lift you to a higher state of happiness, allowing you to enjoy your new routine and your sense of achievement. This can do wonders for your self esteem and general happiness.

Week 7 checklist:

- What type of exercise or activity most interests you? Do some research into the available options in your local area.
- How can you commit to incorporating more movement into your week? What needs to change to make this happen?
- How can you further modify your daily intake to be more support-ive of your exercise? For some of you, this goal may have already

been achieved as your diet is now at its optimum.  For others, maybe it's something simple like having an afternoon snack so that you finish your day with energy to spare.

- Finally, what considerations do you need to make in order to set your SMART or SMARKT goals?  For example, do you need to begin with gentle walking or stretching so that your body is not overwhelmed? Do you get nervous in new situations? If so, maybe commit to going and watching the class or activity first before joining (you could always change your mind and join in when you get there if you feel ready).

X

# Week 8: A low-tox life

# Detox Your Life

Throughout this program, we have addressed many fundamental pillars of health. We've worked on achieving a healthy balanced diet, have reduced our exposure to toxins, optimised our digestion, corrected our sleeping habits, improved our exercise regime and taken measures to reduce stress.

Hopefully, by now, you're feeling like a new you. However, there is another step to take before we finish up. We must discuss the important issue of detoxing our lives and homes.

## Why we need to detox our homes and lives

What you are about to read are some frightening statistics and numbers which really help to bring home how important it is for us to move towards natural products ASAP. There are many areas which we do not have any control over, such as the industrial pesticides used in our local environment, heavy chemical-laden cleaning products which are used on many of the surfaces which we touch each day, the fragrance-filled air which we breathe any time we enter a bathroom or a shopping centre.

However, there are literally thousands of chemicals in our home which we have absolute control over. We can choose to substitute these products for natural products and cut out thousands of chemicals that we are usually exposed to every single day.

In this section, I aim to make you aware so that you can make better, more informed choices. You'll find more resources at www.sydneycitynutritionist.com.

We're going to discuss where the risks lie, the top 10 most commonly used and profoundly toxic beauty products we use every day and how to replace them with practical, natural, chemical free and inexpensive options. We'll then discuss how to remove the chemicals from your home, taking care of your health while also, surprisingly taking care of your wallet. Finally, we'll discuss toxic relationships, and I'll conclude by giving you the end to 21yr old Jen's story.

So without further ado let's get started, shall we?

# Beautiful Poison

It may come as a surprise to you that it is estimated that we are exposed to somewhere between 150 to 500 chemicals every day through our personal care products. It is estimated that there are 13,000 chemicals in cosmetics and only 10% of these chemicals have been tested for human safety.

A study by the Environmental Working Group found that blood and urine samples of teenage girls were contaminated with 64% of the analysed chemicals from four major chemical families: phthalates, triclosan, parabens, and musks. These chemicals are incredibly toxic and have been linked to many dangerous conditions including hormonal imbalances and even cancer.

It is estimated that the average female uses somewhere between 12-16 personal care products every day. Oh and guys, before you tune out here, while the volume of chemical-laden products used each day is higher in females, you are not getting off scot-free either. From parabens and aluminium in deodorants to sodium lauryl sulphate, phthalates, fragrances and titanium dioxide nanoparticles. Our shampoos, body wash, toothpaste, colognes and perfumes are toxic ticking timebombs and we're lathering up daily without a care in the world.

Here's the most frightening statement from the Environmental Working Group:

"Federal health statutes do not require companies to test products or ingredients for safety before they are sold.  As a result, nearly all personal care products contain ingredients that have not been assessed for safety by any responsible agency, and that are not required to meet standards of safety. To protect the health of teens and all Americans, we recommend action."

What's more, the environmental defence group analysed favourite makeup brands and found that a whopping 96% contained lead and 20% contained arsenic. These are products that many of us are using daily and they contain known poisons. In a talk on women's health, I once asked the crowd if they would like to spend the day sucking on a lead pencil. Unsurprisingly, not one person volunteered, and yet we are lathering our skin and lips with these known toxins. Licking our lead-laden lips like we don't have a care in the world.

And it's not just our own health at risk:

A few years ago I attended an annual conference called the International Congress of Natural Medicine. This is a really great conference which I try to participate in every year. It reinvigorates me, energises me, inspires me, and I get to keep up to date with the latest scientific advances in health care.

At this particular conference, however, I spent the weekend appalled and shocked to the core to hear some of the news, research and insights that were shared about how increasingly toxic our world is becoming. I left each day with a growing fierce determination to spread the message of what I had learned. Maybe I knew that one day I would write this book to share the message with you.

The most memorable and shocking story was that of a scientist, who decided to analyse the breast milk of his wife, who was at that time breastfeeding his son. The toxicology report was so grim that he was not legally allowed to pour the breast milk down the sink of his lab. It had to be disposed of as toxic waste! This was the same breast milk that was being drunk by his own son. Scary stuff huh?

But while the level of toxicity here was shocking news, it's not at all uncommon. We have known for years that chemicals are able to be transferred via breast milk and in fact that this is the most effective way for a woman to detox. However, this particular case really brought home the incredible need for a massive transformation in the way we approach our health and well-being programs.

You see, we are living in such an incredibly toxic world now, it is just not enough to follow a standard healthy diet (although, of course, this is a good start). Sadly, however, much of our excellent work achieved with a healthy diet and regular exercise is going to be undone by the chemical cocktail which we are exposed to each and every day. As a currently pregnant female, this is one of my most significant concerns.

## So what do we do about it?

Clearly, there is a need for change. However until this is achieved, it is on us (literally... get it?.. sorry bad joke) to make better choices for ourselves. Take an opposing approach and assume that all chemicals are unsafe until proven otherwise.

There are areas that we have no control over, unless we all pack up our city dwelling lives and live in a permanent eco retreat. However, there is much we can do to reduce our exposure at home.

Now I'm not supposing that you stop washing your hair, brushing your teeth or that you start dragging yourself through a rosebush daily to freshen up (ouch). However I would like to stress the importance of taking measures to clear out all unnecessary chemicals from your life by switching to natural products. It's easier than you might think.

Take a look at my list of the 10 most commonly used, chemical laden, personal care products and their alternatives in my "Swap this for that" cheat sheet coming up next.

You'll be amazed at how easy it is to go chemical free, it's just about taking it step-by-step so that it doesn't feel overwhelming. Replace each item as it runs out with a healthy, natural, chemical-free alternative. You'll have a healthy, happy home before you know it and you'll be saving tonnes of money too.

# Swap This for That Cheat Sheet

Toothpaste

- Often contains titanium nanoparticles which are potential carcinogens (cancer-causing), are linked to Crohn's disease and are incredibly harmful to beneficial bacteria (posing a threat to the health of our good bacteria in our guts, and the bacteria in our environment once excreted).  This newly discovered chemical exposure is currently being studied to determine the exact threat it poses to our health via consumption and to the health of our planet.
- Contains Fluoride which may block iodine absorption leading to (or exacerbating) hypothyroidism and therefore contribute to weight gain, fatigue, constipation and goitre.  Fluoride is not a necessary nutrient and, though it assists with building healthy teeth and bones, the amounts we need are microscopic. With the volume of fluoride in our water and toothpaste, we are building up toxic levels.
- Typically contains sodium lauryl sulphate (SLS) which more than 16,000 studies have determined may cause: cancer, mutations, hormonal imbalances, organ toxicity and reproductive toxicity. Other names for SLS include Sodium dodecyl sulphate, Sulfuric acid, monododecyl ester, sodium salt, Sodium salt sulfuric acid, monododecyl ester sodium salt sulfuric acid.
- Also contains triclosan which studies suggest promotes cancer-causing bacterial growth, development of antibiotic-resistant

bacteria and, again negatively affects the thyroid.

Swap:

- Try using a natural, flouride, triclosan and sodium lauryl sulphate free toothpaste such as Grants which is made from all natural ingredients. This is available at supermarkets for just $3 - $5

## Facewash

- Typically contains SLS which may cause cancer, mutations, hormonal imbalances, organ toxicity and reproductive toxicity.
- Contains parabens which are hormonal disruptors which mimic oestrogen and are associated with increased risk of breast cancer. Parabens are absorbed through the skin and have been found in the biopsy of breast cancer tumours.
- Can contain formaldehyde and formaldehyde-releasing preservatives which are carcinogens (cancer-causing chemicals).
- The chemicals listed above are in most commercial facewash formulas, including those that state they contain organic ingredients or fruit extracts. These chemicals have been linked to cancers including breast, prostate, nasal and nasopharyngeal cancers and may interrupt male reproductive functions.

Swap:

- Try natural products such as Manuka Biotic Face Cleanser or Black Chicken Cleanse My Face Oil. I use the latter, and just a few drops goes a long way. My skin feels and looks fabulous, and you get a free aromatherapy treatment with every wash thanks to the essential oils. This is an excellent choice for sensitive skin, however, do be mindful to transition slowly if you have problem skin. Ideally using the new product once every second day for a week or so to allow your skin time to settle.

## Toner:

- Contains parabens which are hormonal disruptors which mimic oestrogen and are associated with increased risk of breast cancer.
- Contains "fragrances" – this term can mean anything up to 4,000 separate chemicals including Phthalates, another hormone disruptor linked to increased risk of breast cancer, endometriosis, early breast development in girls, and reproductive birth defects in males and females.
- Contains isopropyl alcohol which may deplete your good bacteria in and on your skin, while also weakening the defensive barrier oils.

## Swap:

- Try a natural toner such as rose water, pure witch hazel or even just splash icy cold cucumber water on your skin, fresh from the fridge, after washing with warm or hot water. Any of these methods will produce the desired effect. Choose the one which best suits you.
- For those who would like a homemade version, try adding a bag of green tea to a mug of water. Allow to sit overnight in the fridge, in the morning the solution is ready to be used as your toner after washing.  Be sure to rinse with cold water afterwards for best results.

## Face moisturiser:

- May contain parabens, hormonal disruptors which mimic oestrogen and are associated with increased risk of breast cancer.
- Phthalates, which are often unlisted as they are classified as "fragrances", are linked to increased risk of breast cancer, early breast development in girls and reproductive birth defects in males and females.
- Titanium dioxide nanoparticles, potential carcinogens (cancer-causing) which are microscopic in size, so can easily penetrate your skin and into your bloodstream.  Potential health risks of titanium nanoparticles include nerve damage, DNA mutations and cancer.

## Swap:

- Extra virgin coconut oil, macadamia oil, johoba oil or almond oil make excellent face moisturisers.
- For best results, steam your face first and then rub 2 drops into the palm of your hands, then massage into the face.
- If you have dry skin, I would recommend applying more, leave to soak for 1 minute and then use a soft towel to blot or brush off the excess.
- A jar of extra virgin coconut oil will cost you around $6 from the health food isle of your local supermarket. As a natural antibiotic, it also works well for problematic skin. However, you can add a drop or two of pure lavender or tea tree for enhanced results. **Note:** Be careful to avoid the eye.
- Other options:  Try Andalou Naturals 1000 roses Beautiful Day Cream, or Black Chicken Love My Face Serum

# Shampoo, Body Wash & Soap

- Often contains phthalates, which are linked to increased risk of breast cancer, endometriosis, early breast development in girls, and reproductive birth defects in males and females.
- Sodium Lauryl Sulphate which may cause cancer, mutations, hormonal imbalances, organ toxicity and reproductive toxicity.
- Contains "fragrances" - this term can mean anything up to 4,000 separate chemicals including Phthalates, another hormone disruptor linked to increased risk of breast cancer, endometriosis, early breast development in girls, and reproductive birth defects in males and females.
- Titanium dioxide nanoparticles, potential carcinogens (cancer-causing) which are microscopic in size, so can easily penetrate your skin and into your bloodstream. Potential health risks of titanium nanoparticles include nerve damage, DNA mutations and cancer.
- May contain Nitro and polycyclic musks linked to hormone disruption and cancer.
- Triclosan, another hormone disruptor linked to cancer, thyroid disruption, hormonal imbalances and skin irritation. May also lead to the development of antibiotic-resistant bacteria.


Swap:

- Dr Bronner's liquid soap,
- Thank You Body Wash,
- Thank You Baby Shampoo,
- 100% Pure Honey & Virgin Coconut Restorative Shampoo

## Sunscreens:

- Contain hormone disruptors such as benzophenone, PABA, avobenzone, homosalate and methoxycinnamate.
- These chemicals have been associated with health complications such as increased risk of endometriosis, altered sperm production and alterations in the reproductive system, thyroid and behaviour according to the environmental working group.
- The toxic effects of chemicals in sunscreens is a considerable concern, given that products containing these chemicals are liberally, and regularly, applied all over the body. Even more alarmingly, many of these chemicals are found in the milk of breastfeeding mothers after use of these products.

## Swap:

- Go for natural products which use zinc oxide as the main UV protective ingredient. This natural product offers excellent UV protection and has no evidence of hormonal disruption.
- Our natural sunscreens are really improving in recent years, and I predict that we'll see them improve further in future years.
- I use Andalou Naturals Age Defying Beauty Balm SPF 30 daily as my sunscreen, primer and foundation in one. It offers excellent protection (even for my pasty white skin) and gives a youthful, hydrated, clear complexion. Best of all, it doesn't block the pours leading to breakouts like so many other sunscreens. It took me a long time to find a sunscreen that I could wear daily without suffering from irritated skin and acne breakouts. This product I've used daily for almost 6 months and I'm highly impressed.
- For body: I use SPF 30 Natural Sunscreen Lotion which I find excellent.

## Notes:

Unfortunately, natural sunscreens don't yet go above factor 30. We all know that some days in Oz, where it's impossible to avoid prolonged sun exposure, some of us need a little higher than that. What I do on a day that a higher sunscreen is necessary, is wear the all natural products on my skin to form a physical barrier, and then use a factor 50 on top. This is not ideal of course, I'd much prefer to just sit in the shade where possible. However, it does mean that the primary products absorbed contain natural ingredients. You may still absorb the chemicals from the factor 50. However, it is likely that your absorption will be reduced which is an improvement.

## Conditioner & Hair Serum:

- Contains phthalates, which are linked to increased risk of breast cancer, endometriosis, early breast development in girls, and reproductive birth defects in males and females. Sodium Lauryl Sulphate which may cause cancer, mutations, hormonal imbalances, organ toxicity and reproductive toxicity.
- Contains "fragrances" – this term can mean anything up to 4,000 separate chemicals including Phthalates, another hormone disruptor linked to increased risk of breast cancer, endometriosis, early breast development in girls, and reproductive birth defects in males and females.
- Contains parabens which are hormonal disruptors which mimic oestrogen and are associated with increased risk of breast cancer.
- Can contain formaldehyde and formaldehyde-releasing preservatives which are carcinogens (cancer-causing chemicals).
- Propylene glycol, a small organic alcohol conditioning agent which is a skin irritant and penetrator associated with causing dermatitis and hives.

## Swap:

- Extra virgin coconut oil, macadamia oil, jojoba oil or Moroccan oil make excellent replacements for hair serum. Use enough to lightly coat the palms of your hands and stroke through the hair.
- As a deep conditioner or hair care treatment, try a coconut oil hair mask, coat the hair and allow to sit for 1hour before washing with your preferred shampoo. Further conditioning is not usually necessary. If you have oily or thin hair, you may need to shampoo twice for best results.

## Body Cream:

- Contains Propylene glycol a classified skin irritant.
- Contains phthalates, which are linked to increased risk of breast cancer, endometriosis, early breast development in girls, and reproductive birth defects in males and females.
- Contains "fragrances" - this term can mean anything up to 4,000 separate chemicals including Phthalates.
- Contains parabens which are hormonal disruptors which mimic oestrogen and are associated with increased risk of breast cancer.
- Can contain formaldehyde and formaldehyde-releasing preservatives which are carcinogens (cancer-causing chemicals).
- Titanium dioxide nanoparticles, potential carcinogens (cancer-causing) which are microscopic in size, so can easily penetrate your skin and into your bloodstream. Potential health risks of titanium nanoparticles include nerve damage, DNA mutations and cancer.
- May contain Nitro and polycyclic musks linked to hormone disruption and cancer.

Swap:

- Extra virgin coconut oil (this little star comes in pretty useful). Keep a jar of this handy, and you have a face moisturiser, hair treatment, body moisturiser and even an oral cleanser whenever you need one. Conveniently it's available at your local supermarket for a very low fee.
- Thank You body moisturiser. If you need a break from oil, prefer a creamy base or are just not a fan of the coconut smell, this one is for you. This moisturiser is all natural, and proceeds from this brand go towards helping sustainability charity projects around the world. So you get to give back while also taking care of your body. Best of all, if you're in Australia, you can pick it up for around $6 - $7 for a decent sized bottle from your local supermarket.
- A favourite of mine in the summertime is pure cacao and coconut butter.

## Makeup:

One of the most toxic items on the list, the chemicals in your make up are, no doubt, about to shock and disgust you. However, don't despair, natural makeup is on the rise, and the quality is better than ever before.

## The environmental defence group in Canada found that:

- 96% of makeup contains Lead, a known cancer-promoting heavy metal which may also inhibit healthy thyroid function,
- 51% contain Cadmium - a known carcinogenic (cancer-causing) which is used in clinical trials to enhance the growth of cancer cells, hormonal disruptor which mimics oestrogen, and negatively

affects brain function.[9]

- 20% contained arsenic – which is well known as an effective poison. Long-term exposure can result in thickening of the skin, darker skin, abdominal pain, diarrhea, heart disease, numbness, and cancer.[10]

The FDA conducted a further study on the heavy metal toxicity of makeup in 2016 and declared that, while these metals are present, they are not in large enough amounts to cause harm. However, it was largely underestimated how frequently a female reapplies lipstick. Also, we must consider the long-term implications of these heavy metals, which build up in our system as we cannot excrete them.

These chemicals and more are linked to conditions such as cancer, asthma, fatigue, depression and anxiety. Widespread use of chemicals within our personal care products is being frequently studied with surprisingly negative conclusions. Yet we are usually left in the dark.

Other chemicals which may be present in your makeup are:

- Propylene glycol a classified skin irritant.
- Phthalates, which are linked to increased risk of breast cancer, en-dometriosis, early breast development in girls, and reproductive birth defects in males and females.
- Fragrances – this term can mean anything up to 4,000 separate chemicals including Phthalates.
- Parabens which are hormonal disruptors which mimic oestrogen and are associated with increased risk of breast cancer.
- Formaldehyde and formaldehyde-releasing preservatives which are carcinogens (cancer-causing chemicals).

---

[9]  https://www.ncbi.nlm.nih.gov/pmc/articles/PMC5187886/

[10]  https://www.ncbi.nlm.nih.gov/pubmed/12897217

- Dr Mercola reviewed common lipsticks and collated a list of those to avoid. Lipsticks in the "to Avoid" list include many favourite brands such as L'Oreal Colour Riche (#410 Volcanic), Maybelline Color Sensational (#125 Pink Petal), CoverGirl Queen Collection Vibrant Hues (#580 Ruby Remix), Revlon Matte (#009 Fabulous Fig) and many more.[11]

## Swap:

Luckily many natural brands of makeup exist, chemical free and enriched with natural, plant-based skin conditioners and minerals which may actually improve your health when absorbed. Here's a list of some of my favourites:

- Inika Organic: a fabulous, all natural, organic, Vegan cosmetic company originating from Sydney Australia. I love their products, and they are definitely my go to.
- Andalou Naturals Age Defying Beauty Balm SPF 30 is my favourite daily BB cream. The best part about using natural products is that your skin becomes so illuminated, you really don't want to put on a heavy foundation. This product works perfectly for primer, foundation and sunscreen all rolled into one.

## Note:

My go to for a year or so for chemical free lipstick has been Burts Bees Lip Shimmer, an all natural lipstick made from 100% natural ingredients, or so I thought. On researching to put together an article on natural beauty products, I discovered that Burts Bees lipstick actually contains titanium dioxide. As we do not yet know the full

---

[11] https://articles.mercola.com/sites/articles/archive/2016/08/31/lead-in-lipstick.aspx

implications of this potential carcinogen, I am currently hesitant to use or recommend any products which list this as an ingredient. This was a very disheartening discovery, and it was a sad moment to throw away this favourite which I'd thought was a safe choice. This just furthers my interest in the continuing assessment of the safety of products which we use frequently.

## Deodorant:

Aluminium which is known to possess genotoxic capabilities (meaning it may damage the genetic information within a cell causing mutation and potentially cancer) may interfere with, and cause changes to, the oestrogen receptor, leading to changes in our hormonal metabolism and regulation.

- Contains parabens which are hormonal disruptors which mimic oestrogen and are associated with increased risk of breast cancer.
- Titanium dioxide, currently being studied to determine it's potential health risks, which may include increased cancer risk.
- Triclosan, a known hormonal disruptor which may disrupt thyroid function (leading to fatigue and weight gain) and reproductive hormones.

## Swap:

- My go-to for deodorant is Black Chicken Axilla Paste. This is without a doubt the best natural deodorant I've come across to date. It smells like cinnamon cake batter and has ingredients so natural and healthy that you could literally eat it. Unlike many other natural deodorant solutions, this product offers all-day odour control. Which was put to the test in the Australian summer of 2016, as I suffered through 40-degree heat and a broken air conditioning unit at my office which the landlord was in no rush to fix. Long, 12 hour days in that heat with back to back appointments were the ultimate test for this product, which kept me fresh despite the conditions (I wish I could say the same for my brain). For this reason, I have decided to only recommend this as a natural swap.

I hope you've found this chapter helpful and begin swapping your chemical laden products as they run out with chemical free, natural alternatives. You could use those which I've listed in this chapter or simply research other options for yourself.

Also, I would like to disclaim that I have done my very best to find the most natural and chemical free alternatives for you. However, it is always wise to do further research into each product as occasionally new chemicals come to light, and product formulas also change.

We have been kept in the dark for way too long. New research will no doubt come to light, and new natural products will continue to rise as the popularity for chemical-free alternatives increases.

# Your Daily Detox Regime

Taking measures to reduce our exposure to toxins is a crucial step in creating better health and happiness. However, we must also take time to ensure that we are supporting our daily detox processes wherever possible.

It's important to know that your body will undergo a daily detox whether you support it or not. Supporting these processes allows the outcome to be more beneficial to your health, reduces the symptoms of detox and prevents common side effects such as liver overload, kidney dysfunction, acne, inflammation, headaches, fatigue, moodiness, cravings and nutritional deficiencies.

There are many delicious foods which help to support more efficient detoxification. Many of these we've discussed throughout the course of this 8 weeks. Today, let's put together a daily detox checklist that you can aim for, to assist in achieving our ultimate goal of Pure Health & Happiness.

Detox boosting foods and beverages:

- Cruciferous vegetables: Support liver detoxification. Examples include Asparagus, Artichoke, Brussels Sprouts, Broccoli, Cabbage, Cauliflower, Collard Greens, Kale, Rocket (Arugula),Rutabaga (Swede) and Watercress.
- Citrus fruits: Promote liver detoxification, contain vitamin C to

support liver regeneration, and support digestive processes for optimum clearance of wastes. Examples include Lemon, Lime, Orange, Mandarin, Grapefruit (this last one is particularly potent).

- Foods rich in Beta-carotene (list in week 1): such as sweet potato, pumpkin and carrot help to remove heavy metals from our body and should be eaten regularly.
- Protein foods: Protein doesn't actually initiate detoxification, however many of the amino acids we get from protein are essential for protecting the liver from damage during detox. Daily protein is essential to support optimum detoxification and recovery.
- Sulfurous foods: Stimulate detoxification and help protect the liver from damage throughout. Examples include Garlic, Eggs, Cruciferous veg, Onions, Leeks, Shallots and Chives.
- Teas: Support detoxification and clearance of wastes through the kidneys and bowel. Examples of detox enhancing teas are Green tea (Liver and Bowel), Dandelion (Liver and Bowel), Nettle (Kidneys).

# Detox Your Home

Now that you've read a little more, you are probably not at all surprised that there is a growing interest in natural products. However, just as it is essential to clean up our personal care products, it is equally important to rid our homes from the unnecessary bottles of toxic chemicals sold to us as cleaning products.

Just think, if each product has somewhere between 10-50 chemicals in it, this means you have hundreds, possibly even thousands, of chemicals in your house at any one time. And they are all completely unnecessary.

In fact, we can clean our homes effectively, efficiently, quickly and cheaply with all natural ingredients. It may surprise you, but you can replace most of the chemical-laden cleaning products in your home with just a few natural ingredients.

Here's what you need:

- Baking Soda
- Lemon Juice
- Apple Cider Vinegar
- Optional: Pure clove, eucalyptus or lavender oil

With just the top three products, you can make a refreshing, powerful cleaning solution that will effectively remove grease, dirt, grime, stains and even mould from all surfaces in the house. There really is no need to have the 3-5 cleaning products each for kitchen and bathroom, the toilet cleaner, surface spray, window and mirror cleaner, oven cleaner, dishwashing liquid, dishwasher powder, floor cleaner, drain cleaner etc. etc.

I'll be honest, I have been incredibly surprised at times to discover how much more effective baking soda and lemon juice is than many toxic chemical formulas (and believe me, I've put them to the test). For really stubborn ovens or greased up glass, cream of tartar does a wonderful job too.

These non-toxic ingredients are not only safe, but they also are highly effective, low cost and you never have to worry about children or pets getting hold of them. They are all edible ingredients (they'd decide they don't like the taste of them long before they could possibly do any damage) unlike toxic cleaners which can be poisonous with just a few drops.

Lavender and clove oils are also anti-fungal so can be used as effective mould-ridders. Just spray some on the affected area and leave to sit for a while. After a good 12 hours or more, scrub the area with the lemon and baking soda mix, and you'll be amazed. Industrial cleaning power with just two simple ingredients.

The apple cider vinegar comes in handy when you have a tea (or coffee) stained sink, a greasy oven pan or any really stubborn stain that needs a stronger, yet natural, chemical reaction.

If you have a blocked drain, pour a decent amount of baking soda or cream of tartar (about 1/4 cup) and allow it to sit there for a minute. After 1 minute, add 2 tablespoons of lemon juice and/or apple cider vinegar. The mixture will froth up, allow the reaction to take place and leave it for a few more minutes. Just rinse with warm water afterwards, and you should find your drain is much clearer.

Using these same ingredients, you can also make a fruit and veggie wash, which rids your fresh foods of chemical residues such as pesticides and harmful listeria. This is a handy tool when you can't get access to organic foods.

Baking soda also makes an excellent replacement for powdered dishwasher detergent. It's not perfect, your glasses can come out a little cloudy. However, they are 100% clean.

You can use baking soda as a tooth whitener, simply sprinkle some onto your toothbrush and brush. I usually do this when the toothpaste is still on the brush as it tastes better this way. There are also great natural tooth whiteners made from coconut charcoal which work very well.

**Note:** Some people do use baking soda as a face wash, but I've heard mixed opinions about this. Baking soda is an alkaline substance, and it has the potential to be harmful to the skin by reducing the beneficial bacteria on and in the skin which require an acidic environment.

Finally, you can take lemon juice in water, apple cider mixed with water (or both) as a digestive enzyme, medicinal boost, right before eating and can use baking soda to ease a tummy bug, acid reflux or constipation. So there will never be any wasted ingredients.

# Toxic Relationships

I t wouldn't be appropriate to finish discussing detox without first addressing toxic relationships. There are many relationships which we may encounter in our lives which deplete our health. Some we, unfortunately, may need to endure, such as the stereotypical in-laws who never have anything nice to say. Others we can free ourselves from, once we've identified them as negative.

When working towards a healthier, happier life, it is essential to take stock of those around you and view changes which can be made. Are you getting the support you need from others? Are you spending your days with people who lift you up, inspire you, encourage you and help you to be the best version of yourself?

A healthy relationship is one which is based on mutual respect and trust. There may be imbalances in certain relationships, such as between a mentor and mentee, one has more to learn from the other, yet the respect and trust must be mutual, no-one is more important.

Toxic relationships can be very harmful to your mental and physical health. There are toxic relationships and highly toxic relationships. We should make efforts to reduce our exposure to toxic relationships wherever possible. If this is not possible, then we must at least acknowledge the behaviour and speak with others for help, while also working on our own resilience so that we experience less harmful effects from this relationship.

Highly toxic relationships are those which we must remove ourselves from as quickly as possible. It is important to know that, though common, this is not 'normal' or acceptable, that this does not go on behind all closed doors, and that you do deserve better. The World Health Organisation reports that 1 in 3 women have experienced some form of physical or sexual abuse from a partner.[12] If you feel you or someone you love may be in a highly toxic relationship, seek help. If you don't feel comfortable or safe talking to your loved ones, there are plenty of helplines and support agencies to assist you.[13]

Some examples of toxic relationships include:

- People who only ever talk about themselves and do not check in to see how you are doing.
- People who put you, or others down, to make themselves feel better.
- A person who makes you feel uneasy in their presence, who encourages you to do things you do not want to do.
- A person who depletes your energy, leaving you feeling exhausted after spending time with them.
- A person who adds unnecessary additional challenges or problems to your life.
- People who speak negatively about or to you when your back is turned.
- People who make you feel insignificant or that your views, thoughts, opinions etc. do not matter.
- People who offer advice which is not helpful, rather than listening,

---

[12] http://www.who.int/news-room/fact-sheets/detail/violence-against-women

[13] www.lifeline.org.au/No_Violence  13  11  14  or  Samaritans www.thesamaritans.org.au - Australia

www.nationaldomesticviolencehelpline.org.uk  and https://www.womensaid.org.uk - UK

www.ndvh.org / www.rainn.org - US

when you are in need.

## Highly toxic relationships include:

- Anyone who is emotionally or physically abusive - making you feel weak, threatened, unsafe etc.
- An unfaithful partner who makes you question your own sanity. For example, someone who tells you that you are "crazy" when you question them about suspicious behaviour or tells you that you are "abnormal" for feeling a certain way.
- Any form of sexual abuse, including from your partner. If you are forced into doing sexual acts that you are not comfortable with, are made to have intercourse when you do not want to, or there is more fear than intimacy in your sexual relationship.

## Domestic violence

The United Nations defines violence against women as "any act of gender-based violence that results in, or is likely to result in, physical, sexual, or mental harm or suffering to women, including threats of such acts, coercion or arbitrary deprivation of liberty, whether occurring in public or in private life."[14]

21 year old Jen was in a highly toxic relationship with a man who was emotionally manipulative and physically violent. Let me just clarify when I say that this was not a man that others would see in the street and fear. This was a man in his mid-twenties who had suffered his own physical and emotional trauma from a very young age, who had experienced many hardships that most would find hard to fathom,

---

[14] United Nations. Declaration on the elimination of violence against women. New York : UN, 1993.

many of which made Jen love him in spite of his behaviour and put up with it far too long. Let's call him Mr X.

Day to day Mr X was outgoing, bubbly, friends with everyone. He was funny and affectionate and spoke openly about his love for "his princess" Jen. Behind closed doors he was controlling, would tell Jen that she was damaged and difficult. Day by day these things wore her down. During arguments, things would escalate quickly. On her 21st birthday, Mr X burned himself with an iron, to prove that he wasn't scared of anything, before smashing up the house and throwing her against a wall, then throwing her on the street surrounded by many (broken) birthday presents.

It took almost 2 years for Jen to realise that she needed to get out. One aggressive attack while on holiday overseas left her bruised, beaten and rescued by hotel security. Still, she thought about going back. Mr X had her believing that every negative action of his was her fault. The standard "look what you made me do" phrase was wearing her down daily.

Jen returned from holiday alone and went directly to her mother's house, sporting black eyes, cuts and bruises. There was no turning back now. Once her mum and stepdad had seen this the secret was out. She was forced to talk, rest, eat, recover, and after regaining some strength, she knew what she had to do. Jen left Mr X and, after some recovery time, moved on to a happier life.

Unfortunately, many of our life experiences are perceived through a filter of relativity. What you believe is normal is based on the experiences of your past, and those around you. If there is someone or something in your life right now who is making you unhappy, take some time to think about what can be done, speak to a friend who supports you so that you can gain some perspective, or speak to an impartial adviser such as a counsellor or helpline.

No amount of abuse, physical, sexual, or emotional is normal or acceptable. You deserve a healthy, happy life. You are not damaged. Someone better will want you.

Many people say that they are grateful for the lessons they have been taught by trauma. I am thankful of mine. They helped me to become a more compassionate person, a more accepting person and one who is passionate about helping others. In early 2018 I began formal studies in clinical counselling so that I can help to effect greater change in those who need it. As a result, I have further evaluated the relationships in my past and can see a clear path to many wrong turns and poor decisions I made throughout my youth that inhibited my health, happiness and personal safety. I try to incorporate what I've learned both here, and through my Buddhist faith, to encourage and inspire others to make healthier, happier choices.

Spend your days with people who lift you up, inspire, encourage and respect you. Those who don't are not worth your time or energy. If there is someone in your life who is even mildly toxic, know that this person is suffering too and this is not about you. However that doesn't mean that you should accept this bad behaviour. In my early years of Buddhism, I struggled to find a balance between acceptance and enabling. My good friend Mary, my Buddhist mentor or "guiding parent" as it's called, explained it well when she said:

> In Buddhism, we accept others with unwavering non-judgement and recognise that poor behaviour is often because they are suffering on a spiritual level. Many negative behaviours are born out of trauma and hardship. However, we must not enable, allow or encourage this behaviour. Doing so only enhances the suffering of themselves and others.

In my lifetime, I have accepted plenty of bad behaviour and allowed others to negatively impact my health, happiness and even my behaviours, personality and goals.  I have made many bad choices of my own accord, we all will, but our positive relationships will help to inspire you to do better.

A positive relationship is one which encourages you to be the best version of yourself, that doesn't mean that there will be open-ended acceptance. There often will be times where you'll need to be challenged, questioned or corrected. You may even need to be told off every now and then. However, as a positive relationship is built on trust and respect, there is no fear or shame in this interaction, you can move on quickly, take on board the advice and, importantly, know that your opinion and feelings are still valued.

It can help, when evaluating your life, to take a moment to note those relationships which are positive and those which are toxic. Spend more time and energy nurturing the positives. Try to minimise your interaction with the toxic. And never, ever, allow highly toxic relationships to endure.

# Week 8 Reflection

T his week we have completed our life-changing 8 week program with a review of the factors which can work against our healthy efforts.

In this weeks information I have provided lots more information, tips and possible changes that you can make to achieve greater health & happiness. Before we overwhelm ourselves with change, let's put things into perspective.

Every one of the tips I've provided throughout this program I have personally implemented, however I certainly didn't do them all in 8 weeks and you're not expected to either. The idea is to bring awareness into all the wonderful ways that we can enrich our health, and to provide enough choice to suit every person's needs.

For you, the most important part of this week may have been to reflect on toxic relationships. Or maybe it was a huge shock to learn that your daily beauty regime is loading you up with chemicals that undo many of your daily healthy efforts. As we close this program please work through whatever is most important and best suited to your personal needs. Remember to set yourself SMART or SMARKT goals to ensure that your journey is achievable and kind to yourself.

When it comes to the chemicals in our beauty regime and household products, remember that unless you are suffering with a major health issue, or are currently pregnant or trying to conceive, the best way is to begin replacing one thing at a time as each runs out. For some there may be items you are hesitant to give up, this is fine also. Any change you commit to right now is still a step in the right direction.

## So let's review

- What products are currently running low that you could replace with healthier, low-chemical or natural alternatives? Where can you buy these items?
- What daily practices could you put in to place to counteract some of the toxic load we are exposed to each day? What do you need to do to make time for these?
- What changes do you need to prioritise in your personal relationships? What support is available for you do make this happen?

# XI

# Post-program health, happiness & achievement assessment

# Closing Note: The Language of Nutritional Medicine

Firstly let me say that I love that you have chosen to spend this last 8 weeks with me so that I could share with you my passion for health and healing. There is so much more that I'd love to share, but this will have to wait for future books.

I also love that we now live in a time where food is finally revered. We are spending more time researching and investigating dietary changes which may enhance our health than ever before. We are discussing the benefits of organic foods, superfoods, therapeutic foods, structured eating, fasting and everything in between.

I can say wholeheartedly that it is a beautiful time to be a Nutritionist and an even better time to be a mentor to students and new graduates of Nutrition and Dietetics. It is such a dynamic, and evolving science at the height of its popularity. I am challenged, inspired and further educated every single day. It's a truly wonderful feeling.

However, all the new and exciting research also leads to a lot of conflicting information so I'd like to clear up a few things before I leave you.

As a Nutritionist, we are taught a solid foundation of nutritional biochemistry, anatomy and physiology, which helps to decipher this information quickly and easily. But for the average person, it can all be far too confusing.

I often explain this in the sense that this background knowledge is like learning the mathematical signs in the equations. Put the numbers 2 and 3 next to each other, and there are numerous possibilities. They could make 5, 1, 6, 23, it's the mathematical sign that helps us to make sense of it. We could also call this the language of nutritional medicine. So where sometimes you may get confused, don't worry, that's what the trained experts are for.

We understand the full "equations". We know the whole story. So we can prescribe different foods and critical nutrients at different times. In this book, I've aimed to give you an overview of the steps to optimum health. It is built on a foundation of knowledge taken from my education, my personal experience and years of clinical experience working with my patients.

What I wanted to finish with here is to introduce you to the idea that our body is a complex, complicated and incredible structure, with its own language and scientific equations that requires an incredible amount of study. Hence, at times, we look at basic principles and necessary explanations, and they appear to make sense. We may be drawn in and begin to believe that what is being said is true, when in actual fact it's just because we're looking at two numbers without the plus sign between them, making it just impossible to calculate correctly.

New science is advancing far beyond our current capacity to understand. This will, at times, cause confusion. What I aimed to do with this book is to break some vital pieces of the puzzle down into relatively simple terms, so that you have the knowledge to change and can understand why you'd like to do so. However, I'd love you to embrace, just as all experts do that there will always be so much more to learn. That's what makes us truly special, never dull, and ever evolving.

## How the language of Nutrition helped me

Learning the language of Nutrition has helped me heal from numerous afflictions, physical, emotional and spiritual. Understanding the physiological consequences of the stressors in my life helped me to learn how to reverse them and create a healthier, happier, more fulfilling life.

There are many lessons I was taught by life, many more taught by my studies, and the rest by my Buddhist faith. I've tried to integrate the lessons learned to provide a daily and ongoing care regime for myself that allows me to be the best version of myself.

My stress in my younger years led to PTSD (Post Traumatic Stress Disorder) resulting in many nutritional and emotional deficiencies. My gut function was terrible, I had food intolerances, overgrowth of candida, a lowered immunity, hormonal imbalances and at one stage was told I would not be able to get pregnant without Assisted Reproductive Therapy (I showed them!).

My studies in health science and Nutritional Medicine have helped me understand health and well-being on a cellular level. Nutritional Biochemistry taught me how to correct physiological consequences of stress, trauma and depression through food and nutrients. Buddhism taught me the importance of peace and love and how to achieve it with meditation and acceptance. With this information I could now use food and lifestyle modifications as my medicine, could put in to practice simple changes that could change my life. There was a lot to rebuild from after decades of poor mental and physical health, however piece by piece I've become healthy and whole again.

I am eternally grateful for the people who inspired this journey and who helped my new life to become a reality. My mother, who helped me move to Australia. My grandmother who showed me how to be bold and never fear anything, including major change at any age. My friends, who supported me and stuck with me even when I had my head in the books and no time to socialise. My partner Riaz for being one of my original mentors and for believing in my potential more than I ever did. Finally my guiding parent Mary, for supporting my Buddhist path.

It is thanks to these people that I was able to regain enough strength to become who I am today and to bring this information to you. I hope that the Pure Health & Happiness method has helped you recover the missing parts of yourself so you can get what you deserve. Pure, uninhibited, Health and Happiness is what I wish for you- nothing less.

# What Next?

Now that we've completed the Pure Health & Happiness program, how do you feel? What have you learned about yourself? How do you think your health and well-being has improved thus far?

We have journeyed through many vital elements of a healthy, happy life. I've shared with you the fundamentals that I work through in consultation with my patients. We've discussed how to eat a healthy diet, how to take it a step further and use food as medicine, how to alleviate stress, how to improve sleep and energy, the role of hydration and exercise, and finally, how to detox your life and home.

This has been an incredible journey. A path which took me many years to discover. I'm pleased you allowed me to guide you through it.

Your health and happiness are important to me. You are important to me. I want you to feel fantastic, alive and well every day. These 8 weeks were just the beginning, where you go from here is up to you. I am always here to help if you would like further assistance.

The journey to better health is never smooth or linear. We tend to zig-zag back and forth a fair bit. Hopefully, however, the tools I have provided will allow you to understand yourself better so that you can nurture and support yourself in a kind and compassionate way.

So be kind to yourself. If you occasionally eat too many biscuits, drink more coffee than water, go weeks without exercising, it's ok. Just remember that the more you do to support your health the more you are generally rewarded. When you drop the ball, pick it back up, dust it off a little and get back in the game.

I am so pleased you chose to spend this time with me. It has been an incredible journey, thank you for taking the time to get to know me and my method.

If you would like a little more one on one guidance, join my Pure Health & Happiness online program or book a Skype consultation at www.sydneycitynutritionist.com. I'd love to have you with me.

For now, I'll leave you with a few of my favourite shots from my time volunteering in Myanmar last year with Exousia Australia.

## Volunteering in Myanmar

This was one of my most treasured experiences as a Nutritionist, and I'm truly grateful for the ability to have achieved this lifelong goal. During our time there we spent our days teaching the fundamentals of Nutritional Medicine to Nursing and Midwifery students. In the evenings we visited an orphanage set up by the founders of Exousia Australia who aimed to provide a safe home, education and basic health care to children who were orphaned, abandoned, or those whose families could not afford to take care of them.

With the second least funded health care system in the world (after Sierra Leone) the health of the Myanmar people is largely reliant on their daily self-care. There are very few doctors (those who can afford to train, usually move overseas to wealthy countries where they can make a better living) and many Nurses (after 2-6 months of training) and Midwives (after 3 years of training) become the primary health care providers of their community/region.

Exousia Australia are working hard to effect change by educating on the simple dietary and self-care practices the Burmese people can incorporate each day to achieve better health and happiness. We discussed everything from basic nutrition to maintain life, to therapeutic (local) foods which can be used medicinally to help prevent and treat diseases.

Unfortunately, due to the little one growing inside me, I was not able to revisit Myanmar as planned this year. It's not wise for a pregnant lady to be in those conditions. I do hope to return one day soon though and continue with this great cause.

If you are looking for a worthy cause to contribute your time or money to. Please take a look at https://exousia.org.au/ where you'll find more information.

For now, I wish you Pure Health & Happiness.

Kindest Regards,

Jennifer May BHSc(NutMed).Adv.Dip.Nut.Med.ATMS.MINDD

**Nutritionist**

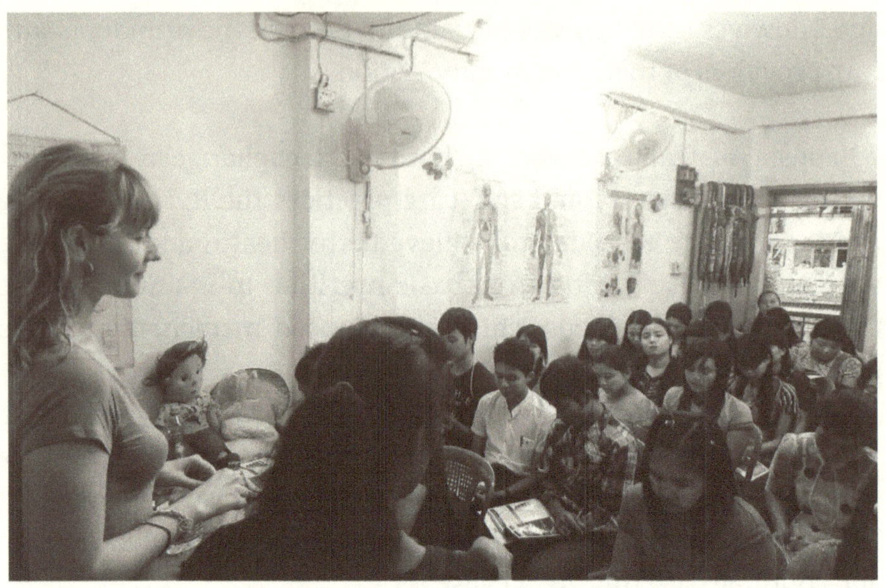

*Our first day in Myanmar. Almost 40-degree heat, a fully packed room and no air conditioning. This was tough after 19 hours of flying and only 5hours of sleep. Hydration was key.*

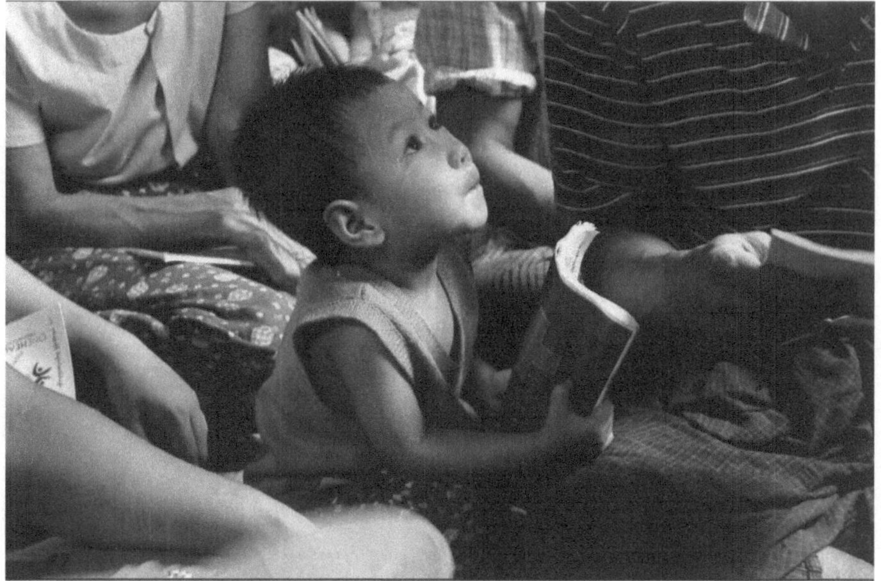

*This gorgeous little guy is a local from one of the villages we visited. Struggling after 2 long weeks of volunteering (and a 3-hour drive in 35-degree heat on rough roads with poor suspension) this is the little face that kept me motivated.*

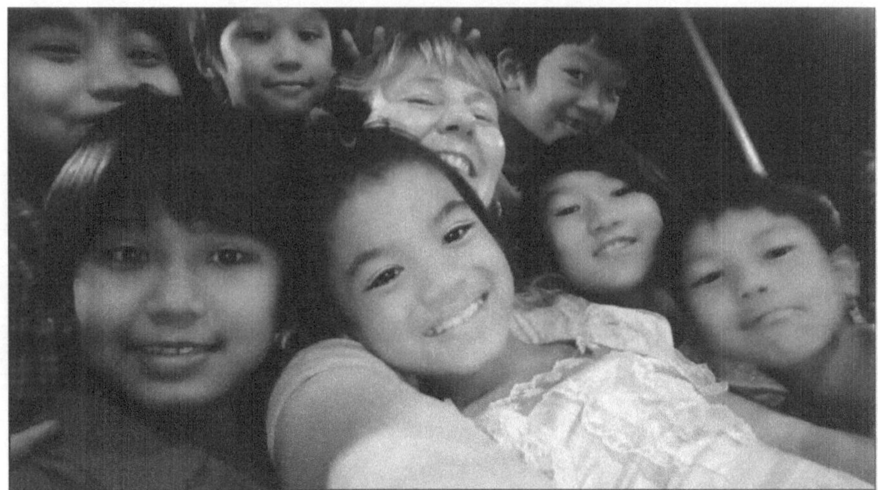

*Here I am swamped with the divine children at the orphanage. There is nothing that can prepare you for the love that you'll receive from these children or the tears you'll cry when you realise the impacts of a simple act of kindness for a child without a family.*

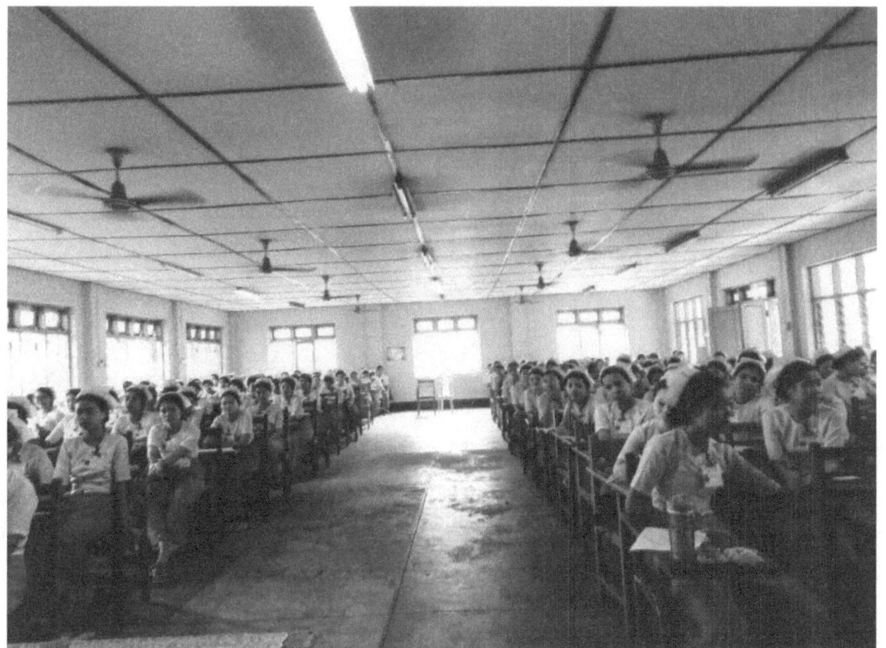

*Our day teaching at the only midwifery college in Myanmar. These ladies will go on to become a crucial part of Myanmar's struggling health care system. I've never met such eager, intelligent, driven and motivated young women. Here we spent a large amount of time discussing women's health, pregnancy nutrition and pediatric care.*

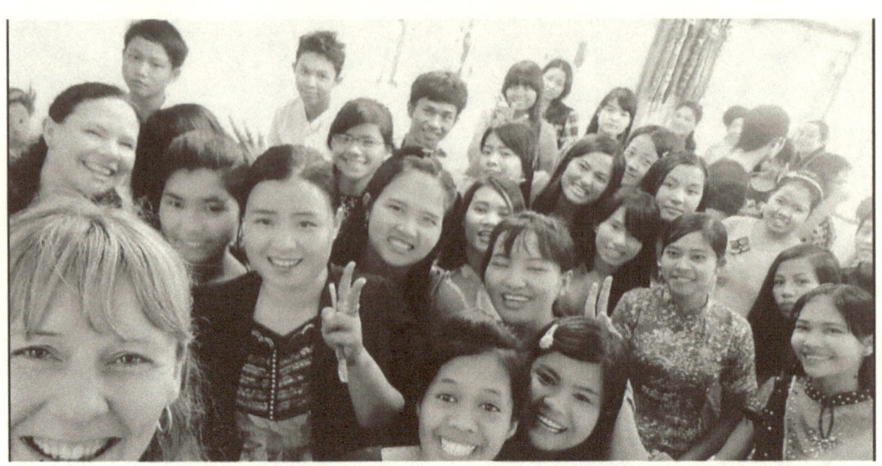

*Lots of happy smiling faces after our first seminar. Feeling hungry, dehydrated, a sweaty mess and dying for a nap . All was forgotten when we saw how grateful and happy these students were, and how much they had learned in just one day.*

# XII

# Recipes

*Here's a collection of healthy recipes which will help you reach the health goals set out in the Pure Health & Happiness program. I apologise for the "real" photos – it was important to me that I'd taken them myself with no professional lighting/Photoshop so that you know exactly what to expect.*

# Healthy Breakfasts

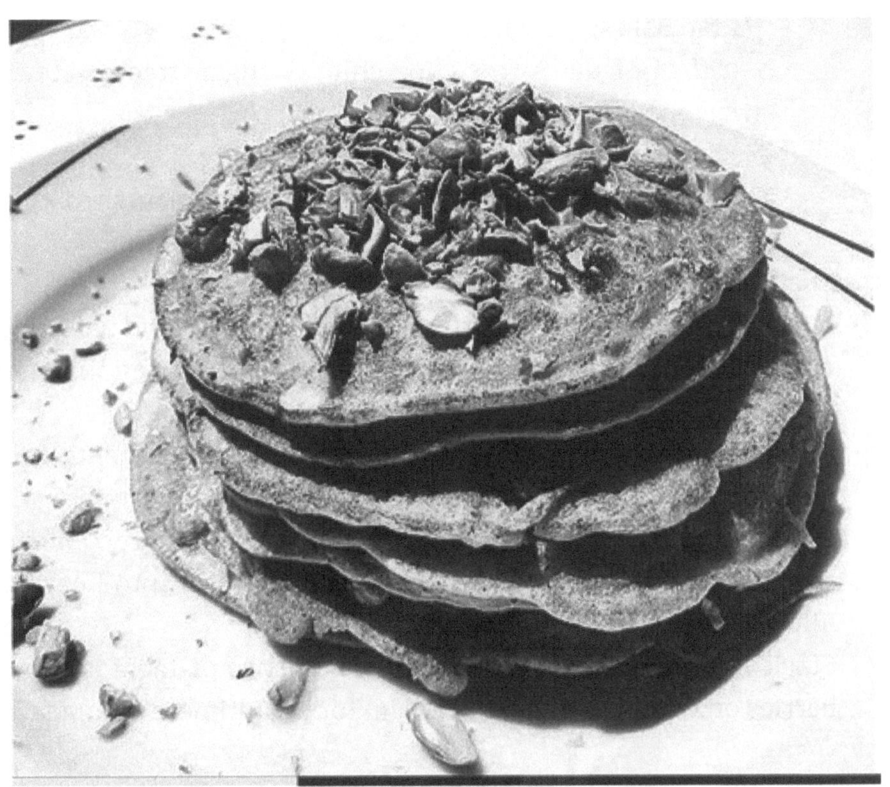

*High protein, high fibre, choc chip pancakes (Serves 2-3. Makes 7 pancakes)*

**I**ngredients:
- 2 cups brown rice flour
- 2 eggs
- 8tsp coconut cream
- 1 tsp balsamic
- 1 tbsp Olive oil
- 1/2 cup rice protein powder
- 2 tsp flaxseed meal
- 4 -5 cups water (until becomes liquid batter)
- 1/2 tsp Baking powder
- 1-2 tbsp of dairy free choc chips - sugar-free or stevia sweetened if possible.
- Non-stick pan or spray olive oil for cooking.
- Optional: 1 tbsp of pistachio nuts, chopped or crushed.

## Instructions:

- Make vegan buttermilk by mixing coconut cream and balsamic vinegar.  Set to one side for 1 minute while preparing mixture below.
- Beat eggs, then add rice flour and all remaining ingredients, mix until forms a smooth batter, now add the vegan buttermilk.
- Heat pan with a little spray oil for best results. Use a cup, or cup size baking measure, and scoop 1/2 cup of batter into hot pan. Allow to cook on one side before flipping.
- Stack your pancakes high.  Dress with crushed pistachios, blueberries or a drizzle of coconut cream for the ultimate indulgence.

* * *

*Flourless Choc-Banana Pancakes for a Serotonin Boost (Serves 1)*

## Ingredients

- 2 eggs

- 1 ripe banana
- 2 tbsp tapioca flour
- 1 tbsp raw cacao or organic cocoa

**Instructions:**
- Blend the banana and egg on high speed for 1-2 minutes to form a light, airy, frothy batter.
- Stir in the tapioca flour and cacao until forms a smooth batter.
- Heat a fry-pan over a medium heat, lightly coated with some coconut or olive oil.
- Pour 1 cup of the batter into the middle of the hot pan. Flip when bottom seems firm to cook both sides. Repeat until all batter is used.
- Serve warm. Best enjoyed alone or with fresh berries and natural yoghurt.

* * *

*Gluten-Free, Paleo Banana Bread (makes 3-4 serves)*

**Ingredients**
- 4 organic eggs
- 3 ripe bananas
- 1 cup of desiccated coconut
- 4 tablespoons of coconut oil
- Optional: You could add 4 teaspoons of coconut sugar, maple syrup or stevia if you prefer a slightly sweeter taste.*

**Instructions:**
- Place all ingredients into a food processor or blender and blend until forms a smooth batter.
- Pour the batter into a loaf tin, lined with baking paper to prevent loss from sticking.

- Bake on 180C for 30-40 minutes.
- You will know when this bread is cooked as the top remains liquid until the very end. When the top is golden and firm, remove from the oven and test by pushing a butter knife from the top to the bottom of the bread - if the knife comes out clean then the bread is ready, if not place back in the oven and repeat after 5-10 minutes.

*I add 4 teaspoons of organic granulated stevia at times, other times I enjoy it with only the sweetness of the coconut and bananas. I'd suggest trying both and seeing which way you prefer it. If going for the sugar option then be sure to serve this with a protein source such as Almond Butter or Tahini.

* * *

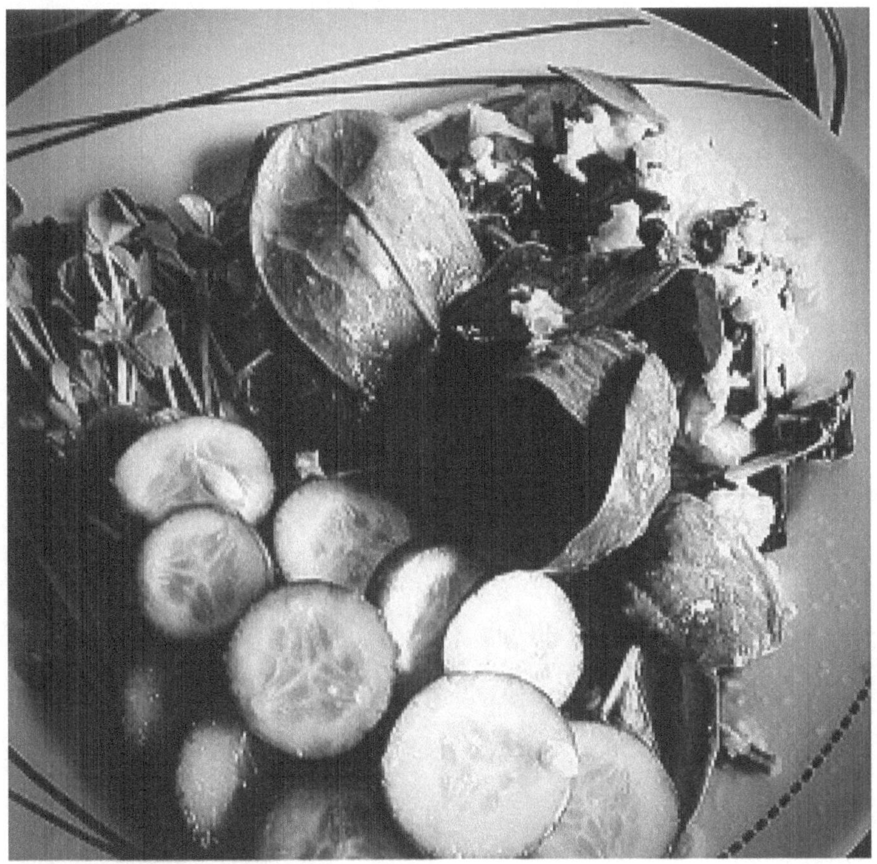

*Super-Alkalising Eggs and Greens*

**Ingredients:**
- 2 Organic eggs
- 1/2 tbsp olive oil
- 3 handfuls of baby spinach
- 1 small Lebanese cucumber
- 1 handful of snow pea sprouts.
- Dressing: 1 tsp extra virgin olive oil, lemon juice (half of a lemon) and a pinch of Himalayan rock salt.

**Instructions:**

- Scramble eggs with spinach and olive oil in a pan over a medium heat
- Load up your plate with sliced cucumber, snow-pea sprouts, and more raw baby spinach.
- Place the eggs in the top corner of the plate and dress with extra virgin olive oil, lemon juice and Himalayan rock salt

* * *

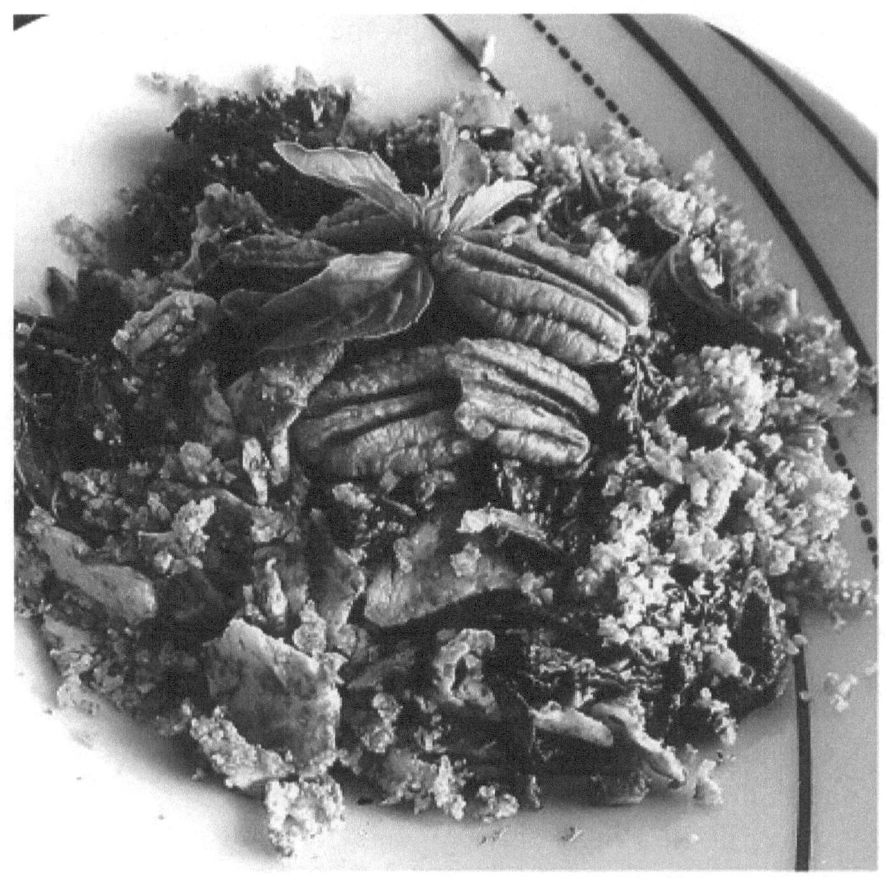

*Pesto Scrambled Eggs with Stir-Fry Greens (serves 1)*

## Ingredients
- 1 large handful of organic kale
- 1 handful of buk choy, chopped
- 2 organic eggs
- Handful of pecans

## Instructions:
- Chop your greens and place in the pan with 1–2 tbsp of your homemade "Super Pesto" (recipe below).  Stir fry for 1minute

before adding your eggs, scramble the eggs with the greens and pesto.

- Take all but 3 of your pecans and grind. I used my magic bullet (the Nutribullet's former, less sophisticated self) for this, but you could use a food processor or even just chop them. Sprinkle 1 tbsp of your pecans over your pesto eggs and greens, place remaining pecans in a jar for other healthy recipes this week.
- Serve your stirfry greens and scrambled pesto eggs topped with ground pecans and a couple of whole pecans on top.
- Enjoy!


*Super Pesto (Makes several serves)*

**Ingredients**
- 2 handfuls of fresh basil leaves
- 2 tbsp pine nuts
- 6 almonds
- 1 handful of kale
- 1/2 cup of extra virgin olive oil
- 3 cloves of garlic
- 2 tsp apple cider vinegar
- Pinch of salt

**Instructions:**
- To make pesto take all ingredients above and blend together using a food processor, good quality blender or simple mortar and pestle. I used my magic bullet which blends everything easily and quickly with little cleanup.
- Place pesto in a jar as you'll need only 1Tbsp for the recipe below with plenty to spare for future inspired creations this week.

* * *

*1 Pot, 5 Ingredient, Shakshuka Style Breakfast (Serves 1)*

**Per Person Ingredients**:
- 1 tin of crushed tomatoes or 2 cups of plain passata (tomatoes only, no additives, read the label to be sure)
- 2-3 cups of kale or baby spinach
- 2 organic eggs
- 1 tbsp extra virgin olive oil
- 1 clove organic garlic

**Super-Simple Instructions:**
- Blend tomato, garlic and oil until smooth.
- Place over medium heat until starts to bubble, stir kale through at this time.
- Crack 2 eggs carefully into the mixture. (I did a bad job of this, but if you're really careful you'll poach the eggs in the liquid which is wonderful.)

* * *

*Multi-Coloured Smoothie Bowl (serves 1)*

**Ingredients:**
- Protein: 1 serve rice, pea, hemp, or grass-fed whey protein
- Colours: 1 cup of multi-coloured Frozen fruit. Tip: purchase fruit that is already quite ripe, chop them and place them in the freezer. Such as banana, kiwi, mango, papaya, pineapple.
- Greens & Bitters: 1 handful of greens - use frozen greens if preferred such as zucchini, spinach, cauliflower or green beans.
- Supercharge: Add 1tbsp of cacao or acai powder to supercharge

this smoothie bowl.
- Toppings for texture: Top with nuts, seeds, fresh fruit and/or a drizzle of yoghurt – see images below for examples.

## Instructions:
- Blend all ingredients together until smooth. Some find a food processor is better than a blender as a blender can leave you with a more liquid texture.
- Top with your chosen toppings (see below for examples).

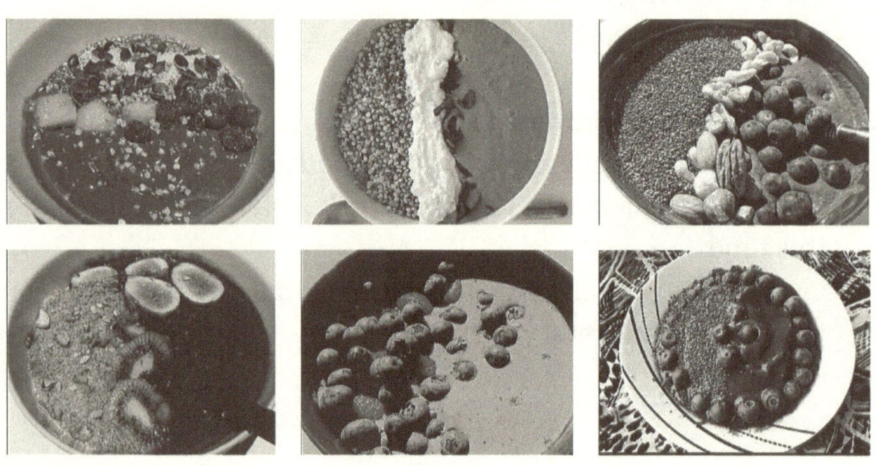

* * *

*Homemade Granola*

## Ingredients
*Granola mix:*
- 1 cup of nut+seed mix – use your favourites. I used a combination of cashews, almonds, macadamias, pepitas.
- 1/2 tbsp of ground cinnamon
- 1 tbsp of coconut oil

*Topping:*
- 2 tbsp of coconut yoghurt
- Handful of fresh berries

*Optional extras:*
- 1 tsp of agave syrup, maple syrup or honey – for those of you who want it sweeter.
- 1/2 cup of rice flakes (Remember, this is optional, you could just double the mix above for a grain free mix or of course use oats if you're lucky enough to tolerate them).

**Instructions:**
- Take the coconut oil and warm in a wok or large fry pan on medium heat.
- Once the oil has melted, add the granola mix to the pan and top with cinnamon.
- Keep stirring the mixture so that it is evenly coated and doesn't burn.
- After a couple of minutes turn off the heat.  If you are using a sweetener such as agave, molasses, maple or honey – this is the time to add it. Drizzle over the mixture and stir well.
- Serve warm and top with coconut yoghurt and berries.

**Notes:**
- If you want to get maximum protein and nutrients out of your nuts I do recommend soaking them for a minimum of 1 hour in water (or overnight) before use.
- Coconut oil is the best oil option for this mix, other options are grapeseed or macadamia oil.
- This mix makes a great breakfast but can also be used as a snack or post-dinner dessert-type treat.

* * *

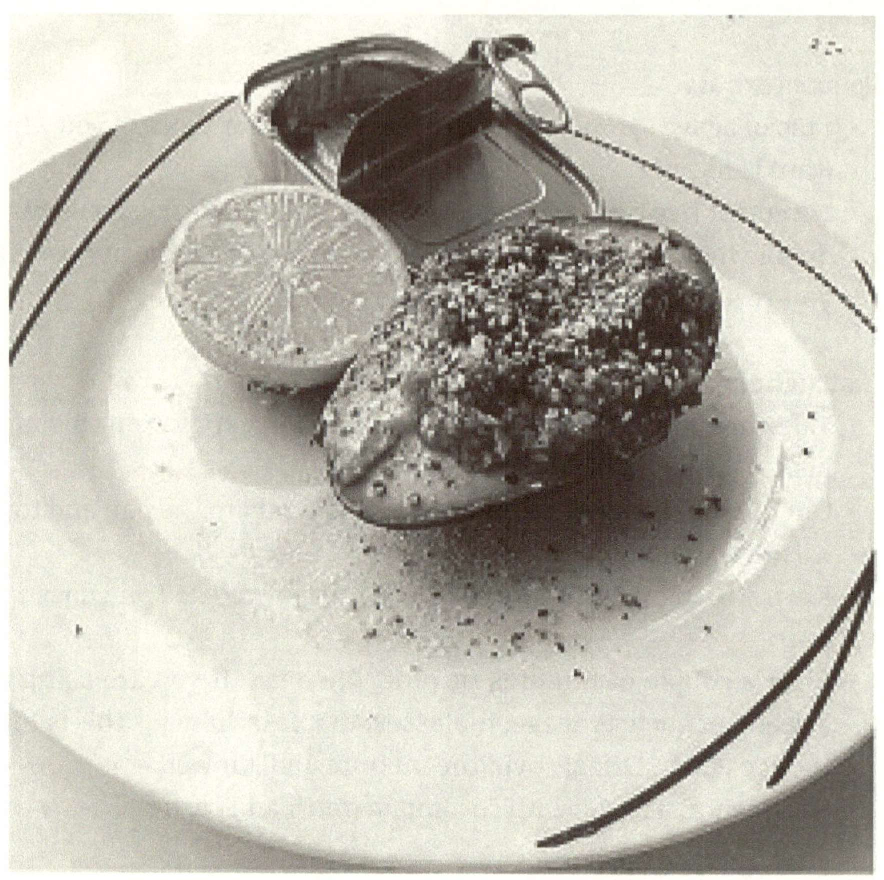

*High Protein Anti-inflammatory, Multi-coloured Breakfast*

## Ingredients

- 1/2 avocado,
- 1 tin sardines
- 1/2 lemon.

## Instructions:

- You could use the sardines in tomato juice as I have here, or the use plain sardines for a very small reduction in carbohydrates (there's only 3g in many tomato versions anyway).
- Scoop the sardines right into the bowl-shaped hole the avocado seed makes, then top with lemon juice. I've also added Himalayan rock salt, cracked pepper and some sesame seeds.

* * *

## Blitz & Go Smoothies

Below is a list of delicious smoothies that you can blend and enjoy on the run on busy mornings. I recommend using an organic rice, pea, hemp or grass-fed whey protein. Please read the label to determine what size the standard serve is and adhere to this guideline. For those with a higher volume of powder per serve, you may find you need to add more water.

- **Choc-Banana Serotonin Booster:** 1 ripe banana, 1 tbsp cacao, 1 serve protein, 1 tsp cinnamon, 1 cup unsweetened almond or coconut milk, 1 cup water.
- **Lung and energy booster:** 1 baby beetroot, 1 tbsp cacao, 1 pinch Himalayan rock salt, 1 tsp raw honey or maple syrup, 1 serve protein, 1 cup unsweetened almond or coconut milk, 1 cup water.
- **Simple rainbow smoothie:** 1 ripe banana, 1 cup strawberries, 1/3rd cup blueberries, 1 handful of spinach, 1 serve protein, 2 + cups water.
- **Alkalising green smoothie:** Juice of 1 whole lime, 1 Lebanese cucumber, 1 cup pineapple, 1 cup lettuce, 1 tbsp coconut cream, 2 cups water.
- **Pina Colada Smoothie:** 1 cup frozen pineapple, 3 tbsp coconut yoghurt (see recipe below for homemade), 1 cup lettuce, 2 cups water.
- **Bircher in a glass:** 15 cashews (soaked overnight), 1 tsp cinnamon,

1 serve protein, 1 grated apple, 1 tbsp flaxseed meal, 2 tbsp coconut yoghurt, 2 cups of unsweetened almond milk.

# Lunch and Dinner Recipes

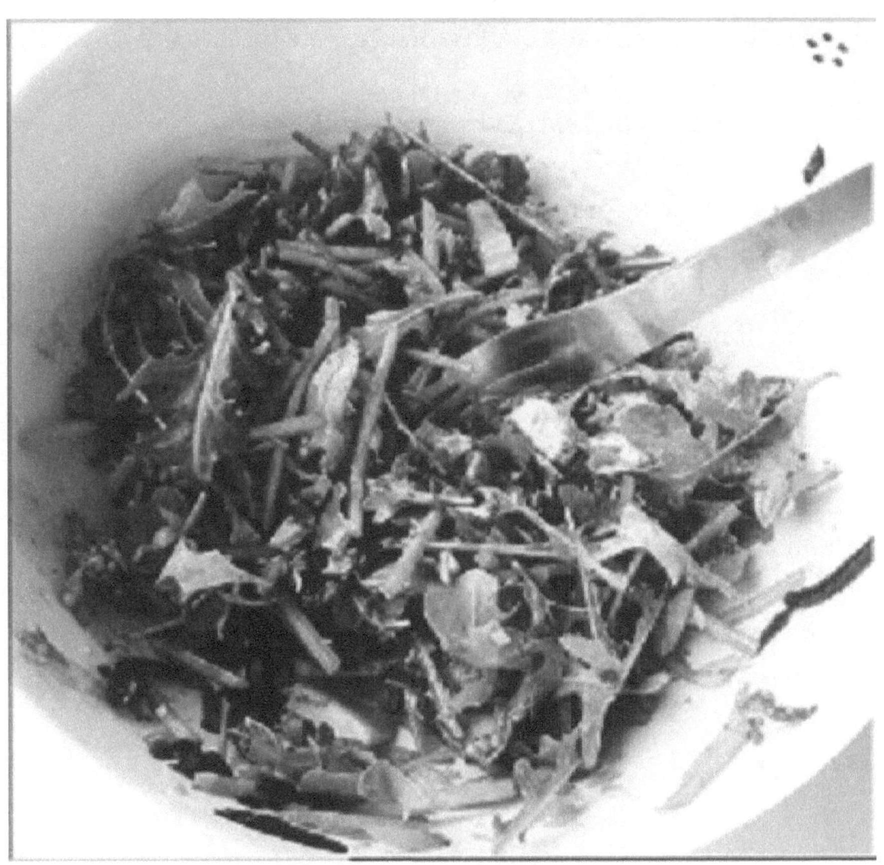

*Rainbow salad (serves 2-4)*

**Ingredients:**
- 2 small carrots, peeled
- 2 Lebanese cucumbers
- 2 1/2 cups shredded red cabbage
- 3 cups of fresh rocket (arugula)
- 2 green onions, thinly sliced
- 80g baby Asian salad leaves
- 50g cooked rice noodles (black or purple rice if you can find it)
- 2 tablespoons extra virgin olive oil
- 2 tablespoons lime juice
- 2 cm piece fresh ginger, finely grated
- Choose your protein:  Boiled eggs, goats cheese or cooked tofu can be mixed through the salad. Beans can be added for fibre, protein and colour. Alternatively, serve with a side of grilled meat or fish.

**Instructions:**
- Slice, grate, dice or spiralize carrots, cucumbers, cabbage, onion, add salad leaves and noodles.
- Mix olive oil, lime juice and grated ginger together in a small bowl. Add to mixture. Toss to combine before serving.
- Serve with a palm size portion of protein.

* * *

*Spicy salmon with Garlic Cauliflower Rice (Serves 1)*

**Ingredients:**
- 100g salmon
- 50g baby spinach

- 1/4 of a head of cauliflower
- Garlic, cumin seeds, chili flakes, black pepper and ground coriander seeds
- 1 tsp of coconut or olive oil

**Instructions:**
- Poach your salmon in hot water for 5-7 minutes or until cooked through.
- Add cauliflower, spinach, garlic, salmon and oil to the pan, stir fry for a couple of minutes, allow the spinach to wilt and the cauliflower and salmon to crisp.
- Add the spices at the last minute, sprinkle extra cumin seeds and chili flakes before serving.

* * *

*Baked fish parcels with hand cut chips and simple salad*

**Ingredients (serves 2):**
- 2 x 100 g white fish such as Basa, Cod or Ling
- Fresh dill
- 1/2 a lemon
- 1-2 cloves garlic, crushed
- Extra virgin olive oil
- 2 cups potatoes sliced in to chip size
- Salt and pepper

**For salad:**
- 1 carrot, grated
- 4 handfuls of green leaves
- Dill
- 1/2 a lemon
- Olive oil

**Instructions, Fish:**

- Preheat oven to 200°
- Take 100 g fillets of fish and place each on foil, ideally lined with baking paper
- Top with lemon juice, garlic, a drizzle of olive oil and pinch of salt and pepper.
- Now sprinkle with lots of fresh dill, wrap into a parcel to allow to steam and then place in the oven.
- Bake for 15-20 minutes or into cooked through. Serve to the table in parcels for maximum effect.

**Instructions, chips:**

- Boil potato until soft in a large pan with water and a sprinkle of salt.
- Once cooked, place in a fry pan with a light coating of olive oil and stir fry until crispy.

**Instructions, Salad:**

- Mix greens, grated carrot, and dill in a bowl.
- Dress with juice of half a lemon plus a drizzle of olive oil.

* * *

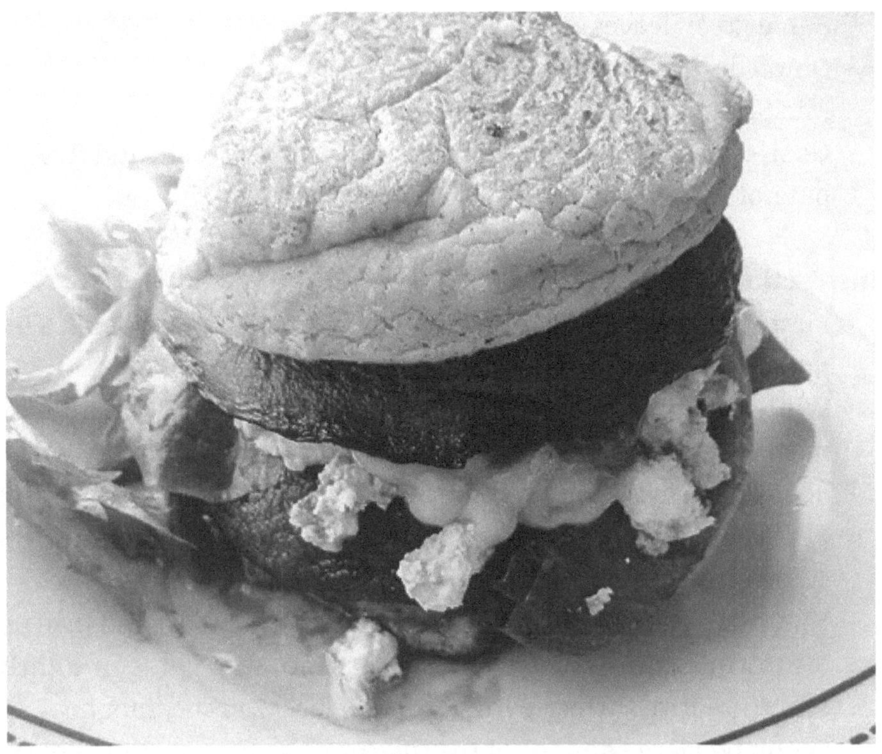

*Field Mushroom Burger in a High Protein Grain-free BeanyBun*

## Ingredients:

- 1/2 of a tin of cannellini beans
- 1 organic egg
- 1 tbsp flax meal
- 1 tbsp almond meal (or quinoa flour if you prefer)
- 2 large field mushrooms
- Salt
- Pepper
- Olive oil

## Garnish:

- Some green leaves
- Onion or tomato relish
- Mustard
- Goat's cheese (optional ingredient for extra protein and flavour but not essential)

**Instructions:**
- First, pan-fry the mushrooms in just a small amount of oil. This lightly cooks them and reduces the water content.
- While they are cooking, blend the egg, beans, flax and almond meal with a pinch of salt and pepper. I used a magic bullet which does this in less than 1 minute.
- Flip your mushrooms to cook the other side - watch out for spitting as the juices hit the oil.
- Now place your mushrooms under urge grill to toast and firm up. Meanwhile, rinse the pan and wipe clean, now spray or lightly coat the entire surface with olive oil. Place over medium heat.
- Spoon two large dollops of the mixture into the pan and allow to cook for 2 minutes. You should see it start to lift and firm, you can also test by trying to nudge or slide them around the pan.
- When firm enough, flip your "buns". The other side should cook in 1-2 minutes also.
- Place the first bun on the plate, stack tall with your mushrooms, greens, mustard, tomato relish, and cheese if you're using it.
- Finish with another bun slice and don't forget to Instagram your work!

* * *

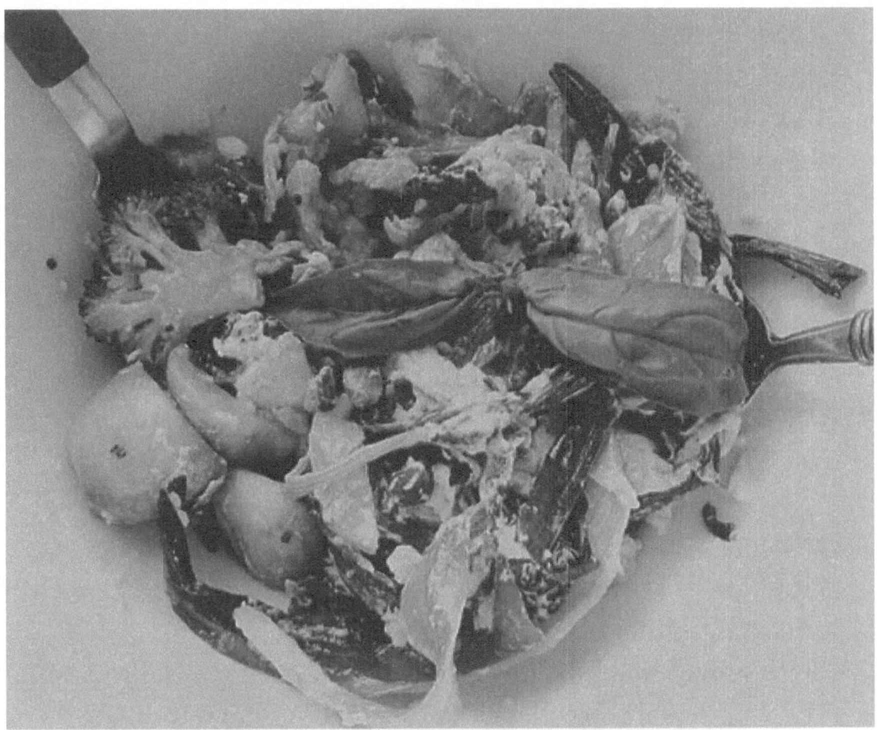

*Stress-Less and Detox with Loodles (Leek Noodles)*

**Ingredients:**
- 1 cup of broccoli
- 1 cup of mushrooms
- 3 asparagus spears, snapped or chopped into bite–size pieces
- 1 handful of basil
- 1/2 a head of a leek, torn into ribbons
- 2 organic eggs, beaten
- 1 tbsp extra virgin olive oil
- Optional: 1 tbsp of goats cheese or a sprinkle of coconut butter

**Instructions:**
- Stir fry the greens in olive oil for 3–4 minutes.

- Add in the eggs as you turn off the heat. Stir well, so the egg cooks among the heated veggies
- Serve with goat's cheese or a sprinkle of coconut butter and stir through.

**Note:**
- For the meat eaters, this would also work well with some chicken chopped through it.
- For the lean and green vegan machines, you can take out the eggs, double the broccoli and top up the fats further by stirring some coconut cream through while cooking.

**Benefits:**
- This dish is rich in vegetarian #protein plus antioxidants and important minerals like iron and magnesium.
- The greens and good fats are great for reducing inflammation.
- The asparagus, broccoli and leek are fabulous for improving detoxification, digestion and can reduce sugar cravings significantly.

* * *

*Spiralised Zucchini Pasta with Fresh Basil & Tomato Sauce*

**Ingredients:**
- 1 zucchini peeled or spiralled into "pasta" sheets
- 1/2 a cup of organic button mushrooms
- 1 punnet of fresh cherry tomatoes
- 1 handful of fresh basil leaves
- 1/2 a cup of crushed tomatoes (from a jar or bottle rather than can if possible)
- 1 clove organic garlic
- 1 tsp of chili

**Instructions:**
- Add all ingredients to a large pan and heat for 2 minutes.
- Turn down once starts bubbling and allow to simmer for 2-3 more minutes
- Season with Himalayan rock salt and black pepper.

* * *

*Healthy Homemade Vegetarian Lasagne (serves 3)*

This dish is perfect for getting a healthy balance of plant-based protein, healthy carbohydrates and lots of vegetables in several different colours.

**Ingredients:**
- 400g cooked brown lentils
- 400g crushed tomatoes or passata
- 1 cup chopped tomatoes
- 1/2 red capsicum (bell pepper)
- 100g chopped mushrooms
- 1 grated carrot
- 2 handfuls of baby spinach
- Spelt, Pulse or Gluten Free Lasagne Sheets
- 1/4 leek torn into long strips
- 1 x red onion
- 2 cloves garlic
- 2 tbsp tomato paste
- 2 tbsp extra virgin olive oil
- Salt & Pepper
- 50g cheese[15]

---

[15] Cheese is typically made with an enzyme removed from a calf's stomach called rennet. If you're vegetarian be sure to use vegetarian cheese which is made from non-animal rennet.

**Instructions: (to make the 'sauce')**
- Preheat the oven to 200 degrees Celcius.
- Place mushrooms, spinach, tomatoes, onions, lentils and garlic in a pan with olive oil and stir-fry for 2 minutes.
- Add remaining veggies (not leeks) and stir-fry for another 3-5 minutes.
- Add the passata/crushed tomatoes and a pinch of salt. I like to add a good grind of pepper here 1 full teaspoon will give it a good kick. Allow to simmer for 5-7 minutes.

**Instructions: (to make the Lasagne)**
- Scoop a layer of sauce into a baking dish. Now add a layer of leek strips.
- Next, add another layer of sauce and a layer of lasagne sheets. Top with a light layer of grated cheese.
- Layer the sauce, then leek, then sauce, then lasagne sheets plus cheese until the dish is full. Top with a layer of sauce and more cheese.
- Cover pan with baking paper and a layer of foil before placing in the oven. It will need to bake for around 35 to 40 minutes.
- Serve alone or with a delicious side salad.

* * *

*Colourful Detox Vegetable and Potato Pie (serves 3)*

**Ingredients:**
- 2 cups chopped potatoes (chop into 1-2cm pieces)
- 400g (or 1 tin) cooked brown lentils
- 400g crushed tomatoes or passata
- 1 cup chopped leek
- 1 grated carrot
- 1 cup finely chopped or grated brussels sprouts

- 1 onion
- 2 large cloves garlic
- 1 cup green peas
- 1/2 cup cottage cheese
- 1 cup grated cheese (optional)

**Instructions:**
- Place potatoes in a small pan to boil until soft
- Heat oven to 200 degrees
- In a large fry pan add leek, onion, garlic, brussels sprouts and 1 tbsp of oil Heat the oil with the ingredients, stirring regularly.
- Add a pinch of nutmeg and four spice and stir to coat all ingredients
- After onions have browned, add carrot and lentils and stir continuously to soften
- Now add crushed tomatoes, 1 cup water and green peas. Allow to simmer until sauce reduces and thickens.
- Once the potatoes are ready, drain and mash. Add a pinch of salt, some pepper and a drizzle of oil. Combine the cottage cheese with the potato now.
- When the sauce has thickened, spoon into a loaf tin (if you have very fussy eaters, you could add to a food processor or blender first to rid the veggie evidence. However be careful with the blender as blending hot ingredients can cause explosions).
- Top with a layer of mashed potato. Then coat with cheese if you're using it. Otherwise a layer of pepper and a little more salt.
- Place under the grill for 5 mins to brown the cheese.
- Serve alone or with a side salad

# Healthy Snack Ideas

*Fresh Berry Treat (serves 2)*

**Ingredients:**
- 1 cup blueberries
- 1 cup chopped strawberries
- 4 tbsp greek yoghurt or coconut milk yoghurt
- 1 tsp raw honey or maple syrup

**Instructions:**
- Wash and dry the berries and place on top of yoghurt
- Drizzle with honey before serving.

* * *

*Immunity Boosting, Multicoloured, Phytonutrient Rich Salsa*

**Ingredients**
- 3 Roma tomatoes
- 1 cup sugar snap peas
- ¼ head of red cabbage
- ¼ Lebanese cucumber
- 1 red capsicum
- 1 small red chili
- 1 small green chili

- Extra virgin olive oil
- Balsamic vinegar
- 1 lemon
- 1 lime
- 3 cloves garlic
- 2 tsp chopped mint
- 2 tsp chopped coriander

**Instructions:**

- Chop all salad vegetables into chunky pieces and mix in a bowl. Finely chop garlic and add to mixture along with mint and coriander. Squeeze in the juice of lemon and lime and stir well. Drizzle 1 dessert spoon of extra virgin oil and finish with balsamic vinegar.

* * *

*Immunity Boosting, Phyto-nutrient Rich Tom Yum Tea*

(think of it as a spicy watery soup)

**Ingredients**

- 1 tsp apple cider vinegar,
- 1 chopped clove garlic,
- 1 tsp cayenne pepper,
- 1 tsp turmeric,
- ½ tsp ground cloves
- 1 tsp chopped coriander

**Instructions:**

- Take all ingredients and add to a tea strainer or teapot mixed with hot water. Allow to simmer for a couple of minutes before drinking.

* * *

## *Homemade Coconut Yoghurt*

**Ingredients:**
- 200g coconut milk (or coconut cream if you'd prefer it thick and creamy)
- 1 capsule of probiotics containing Lactobacillus and Bifidobacterium
- 1 clean and empty jar

**Instructions:**
- Add the coconut milk to the jar, split the probiotic capsule open and pour in the powder. Stir well to combine.
- Place a clean tea towel or muslin cloth over the jar in place of a lid, secure with an elastic.
- Place the jar in the cupboard overnight. Smell and taste in the morning - if it smells and tastes sour, it is ready - screw on the lid and place in the fridge. If you prefer a stronger taste, place back in the cupboard.
- Note: If it is a particularly warm day the yoghurt may ferment more quickly.
- Serve with fresh berries, add to smoothies, or mix with lime juice for a yoghurt salad dressing.

* * *

## *Black Bean Hummus & Veggie Sticks*

**Ingredients:**
- 200g cooked black beans
- 1 clove garlic
- Juice of 1 lemon

- 1 tbsp raw pine nuts or hemp seeds
- 2 cups of chopped raw veggies such as capsicum (bell pepper), celery, carrot, cucumber.

**Instructions:**

- Blend all ingredients (except veggies) until smooth
- Enjoy as a dip, dressing, side etc. for a protein, fibre and healthy carbohydrate boost.

# Healthy Indulgence

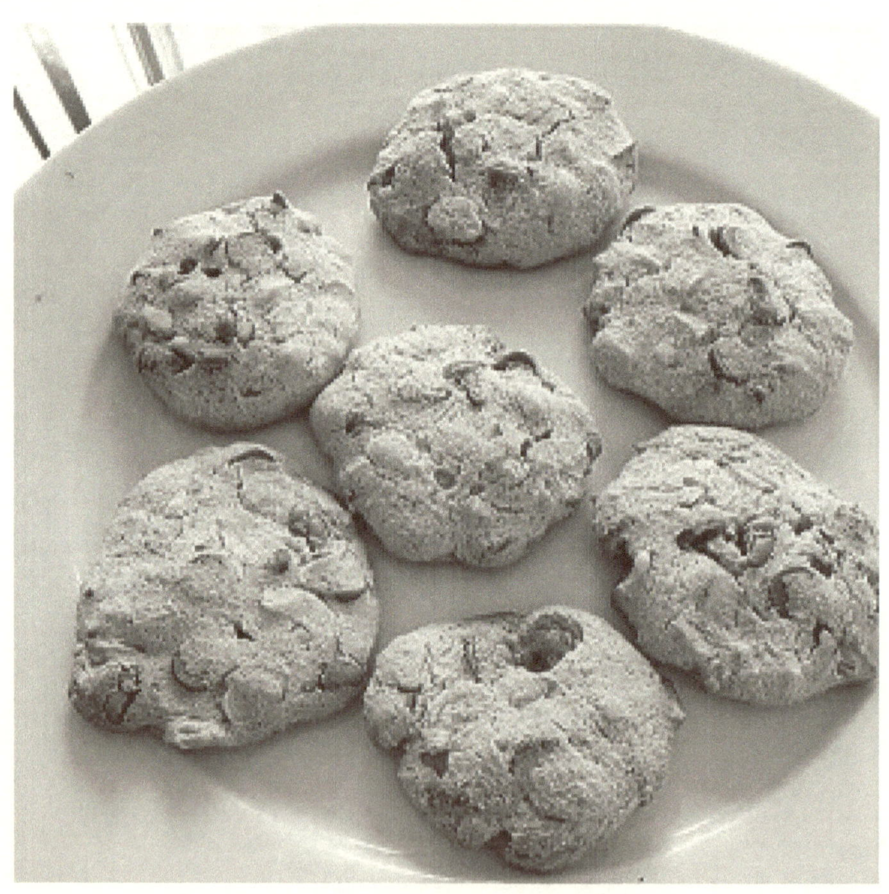

## High Protein Choc-Chip Cookies

**Ingredients:**
- 1 tbsp coconut oil or organic butter
- 1 egg
- 2tbsp chopped homemade chocolate (see recipe below) OR naturally sweetened chocolate chips
- 4 tsp organic stevia
- 3 heaped tbsp of protein powder – I used Vital Greens Vital Protein (vanilla flavour)
- 2 tbsp chopped raw nuts – I used almonds, macadamia nuts and walnuts

**Instructions:**
- Pre-heat the oven to 200 degrees
- Mix protein powder, egg and stevia together in a bowl. Mix well until it forms a sticky dough.
- Now add the coconut oil and keep stirring until has mixed through.
- Add the choc chunks and chopped nuts now, stir or knead the dough until is evenly dispersed.
- Grease a cookie tray or line with baking paper to prevent from sticking.
- Take sections of the dough and roll into balls, pat down onto the tray leaving around 1cm between each cookie. These cookies won't spread much, so they don't need too much extra space.
- Bake on 200 degrees for 15-20 minutes or until golden brown. Keep checking and take them out when edges start to crisp.
- Take them off the tray and let them cool for 20 minutes or so – this is important as these cookies, given the lack of flour, will have a strange, spongy texture until cooled. However, once they have cooled, they will be crunchy yet just chewy enough to make them indulgent. The choc chips and crunchy chopped nuts are a delicious combination.

* * *

*Blueberry Chocolate Bar*

**Ingredients:**
- Take 1 tbsp of raw cacao
- 1/2 of a cup of coconut milk
- 3 tbsp coconut oil or macadamia oil
- 1 punnet of fresh blueberries
- Option: For the sweetener, add 2 tsp of stevia, honey or maple syrup. Personally, I like it without the sweetener.

**Instructions:**
- Line a plastic container with some baking paper – this helps with removing the chocolate later.
- Lay the (washed) berries out across the bottom of the container now. Be sure to spread them evenly.
- Place a pan of water over medium heat and bring to the boil.
- Once boiling, add a bowl to the boiling water – very carefully.
- Take the oil and cacao and mix together in the heated bowl until melted. Keep stirring to avoid burning.
- Once you have a melted chocolate mixture, add the coconut cream and stir well. Carefully taste the mixture to see if you need to add the sweetener.
- If needed, add the sweetener now and remove from the heat while continuing to stir.
- Pour the melted chocolate mixture into the container, if using berries, be sure to cover them evenly.
- Place in the fridge for 1hour to set. If not using berries, you could place in the freezer to set more quickly.
- Enjoy with a cup of green or white tea. Share with friends if you are feeling generous.
- Note: this chocolate is highly energising. Consume earlier in the

day.

* * *

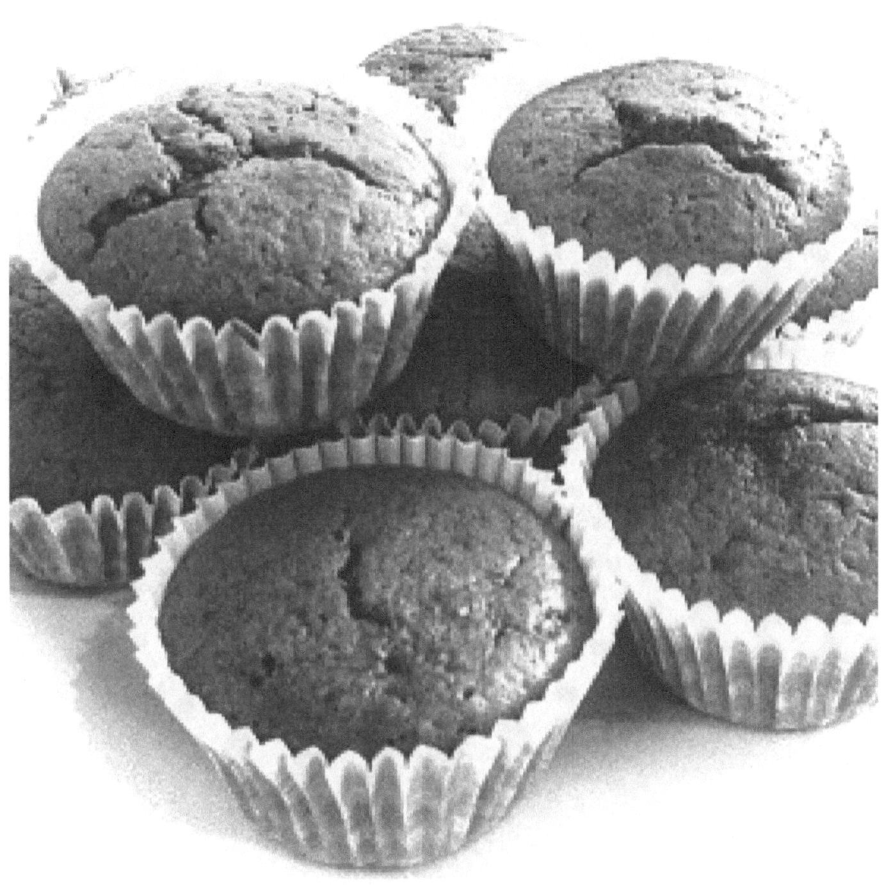

*Healthy Homemade Chocolate Muffins*

**Ingredients**

- 3 organic eggs
- 1 cup coconut cream
- 1 cup coconut sugar (or 1/2 a cup of organic granulated stevia)
- 1.25 cups quinoa flour
- 1 cup raw cacao
- 2 tsp vanilla bean extract
- 1 cup coconut oil
- 1/2 tsp baking soda
- 1/2 tsp baking powder
- 1/2 tsp Himalayan rock salt

**Instructions:**

- Preheat oven to 200 degrees Celcius.
- Mix all dry ingredients together in a bowl.
- Add wet ingredients and mix well.
- Pour mixture into lined or greased muffin tray and place in the oven for 25–30 minutes (check occasionally as oven times will differ).
- To test – place a knife into the centre of a cupcake and poke to the bottom. If the knife comes out clean when you remove, then the cupcakes are ready.

* * *

*Indulgent Vanilla Choc-Chip Protein Muffins*

**Ingredients:**

- A small pinch of salt
- 1/3 cup of coconut sugar
- 1/2 cup of organic granulated stevia
- 1 tsp bicarbonate of soda
- 1 cup of millet flour
- 1 cup of water

- 1 organic egg
- 1 tbsp apple cider vinegar
- 1/3 cup of vanilla pea protein
- 5 tbsp liquid coconut or macadamia oil
- 1 tsp xantham gum
- 2 tbsp chopped chocolate chunks (here I used chunks of my own homemade vegan chocolate. However, you could use any of your favourite chocolate)

**Instructions:**
- Preheat the oven to 180degrees
- Mix all dry ingredients (not chocolate chunks) together in a bowl until evenly combined.
- Mix all wet ingredients together in a separate bowl until evenly combined.
- Add wet ingredients to dry ingredients and mix gently until smooth batter forms. Add chocolate chunks here and mix until evenly spaced.
- Bake in the oven for 20-30 minutes, checking occasionally. Muffins are cooked when you can poke with a toothpick all the way to the bottom and remove clean.
- Enjoy with a cup of your favourite tea!

* * *

## Choc-Avocado Pudding

**Ingredients**
- 1 whole avocado
- 1 tablespoon organic cocoa or raw cacao
- 1 teaspoon of agave nectar or manuka honey
- 1 tablespoon chia seeds (optional)

**Instructions:**
- Take all above ingredients and mix well until mousse-like texture.
- Serve alone or topped with a few berries

**Variations**
- If you're not trying to lose weight, a banana works very well mashed into this recipe. This works particularly well when preparing for Children. If you're working on a weight loss program however then it's best to keep it simple - maybe try the spicy option below instead.
- For an extra creamy treat, or to make it slightly more filling, you could also add 1 tablespoon of coconut yoghurt or coconut cream
- For an extra fat burning, metabolism boosting, spicy treat, try adding 1 teaspoon cayenne pepper or ground chili. Note: This option does add an additional metabolism boost, and choc-chili is quite delicious but remember spice isn't for everyone - use only if you enjoy.

* * *

*Healthy Homemade Blueberry Muffins*

**Ingredients**
- 3 organic eggs
- 1 cup coconut cream
- 1 cup coconut sugar (or 1/2 of a cup of organic granulated stevia)
- 1.25 cups quinoa flour
- 2 cups of blueberries
- 2 tsp vanilla bean extract
- 1 cup coconut oil
- 1/2 tsp baking soda
- 1/2 tsp baking powder
- 1/2 tsp Himalayan rock salt

## Instructions

- Preheat oven to 200 degrees Celcius.
- Mix all dry ingredients together in a bowl.
- Add wet ingredients and mix well.
- Pour mixture into lined or greased muffin tray and place in the oven for 25-30 minutes (check occasionally as oven times will differ).
- To test - place a knife into the centre of a cupcake and poke to the bottom. If the knife comes out clean when you remove, then the cupcakes are ready.

# Healing Real-Food Teas & Drinks

*Sleepy Detox Tea*

**Ingredients:**
- 1 bag of dandelion tea
- 100-200ml unsweetened almond or rice milk
- 1/4 tsp of honey
- 1/4 tsp of cinnamon

**Instructions:**
- Brew the black tea with hot water until it forms a deep brown colour.
- Now add the cinnamon and stir well before adding the milk and touch of honey.
- Sip slowly and enjoy

* * *

*Tom Yum Tea - For a powerful detox and immunity boost*

**Ingredients:**
- 1tsp apple cider vinegar,
- 1 chopped clove garlic,
- 1 tsp cayenne pepper,
- 1 tsp turmeric,

- ½ tsp ground cloves
- 1 tsp chopped coriander

**Instructions:**

- Take all ingredients and add to a tea strainer or tea pot mixed with hot water. Allow to simmer for a couple of minutes before drinking.

* * *

### Easy Cold & Sore Throat Cure – Garlic Tea

Garlic is natures anti-biotic, increases white blood cell production and can quickly bring down a fever. It's pungent flavour can also help to clear the sinuses and sooth a sore throat but be sure to have a jug of water ready as it will make you thirsty.

**Ingredients:**

- 1-2 cloves of garlic
- Boiled water

**Instructions:**

- Take garlic and chop roughly. Add to hot water and allow to simmer for 1-2 minutes before serving.

* * *

### Turmeric, Ginger & Honey Tea

**Ingredients:**

- 1/2 tsp ground turmeric
- 1 tsp crushed or sliced ginger
- 1/2 tsp raw organic honey (manuka honey is best if you can get it

- Boiled Hot water
- Optional: 1 tbsp of unsweetened coconut cream

**Instructions:**
- Add turmeric, ginger and honey to hot water and stir well to combine.
- Add coconut cream (if you're using it) and stir well.
- Sip slowly and breath deeply. Enjoy the antiinflammatory, mood boosting effects of these ingredients. This tea is well suited to any time of day.

* * *

*Super Indulgent Hot Chocolate*

**Ingredients:**
- 1-2 tsp organic cocoa or cacao
- 1-2 tbsp coconut cream
- Hot water
- 1 tsp of molasses or pure honey
- Optional: 1 tbsp of cacao butter (this is optional but does make it more of a rich, melted chocolate drink, rather than cafe style hot chocolate. However be mindful that along with all the beneficial fats, this adds a lot of calories.)

**Instructions:**
- Grate the cacao butter if you're using it so that it melts easy. Add to a cup and pour hot water - stir well to mix.
- Add the cocoa/cacao powder now, stir through until mixed well.
- Add the molasses/honey and continue to stir.
- Finally, add the coconut cream.
- Sip slowly and thoroughly enjoy every mouthful.

# Thank You & Resources

Thank you for joining me on this journey to Pure Health & Happiness. I hope that you have found this book as inspiring as it is informative.

To assist you in your journey I have resources available for download at www.sydneycitynutritionist.com/PureHealthAndHappinessBook

If there are any particular resources which you feel you'd like to see in future, or if you have any feedback on how this book assisted your recovery, please email me at info@sydneycitynutritionist.com.

For those who would like some personal, one on one guidance, or would benefit from a detailed health overview with tailored advice, consider my Comprehensive Health Screening. You'll find this, and many other healthcare services at my business website https://www.sydneycitynutritionist.com/shop. Also watch this space for the Pure Health & Happiness online program which is coming up soon.

Finally, please remember that your feedback and support is greatly appreciated and will determine the success and reach of this book, and those which I intend to write in the future. Please do remember to leave me a review on Amazon. Your honest review will help others to determine if my guidance is right for them.

www.ingramcontent.com/pod-product-compliance
Lightning Source LLC
Chambersburg PA
CBHW051038250726
48656CB00001B/23